Unleashing the Power of Onions

Harnessing the Healing Properties of Onions

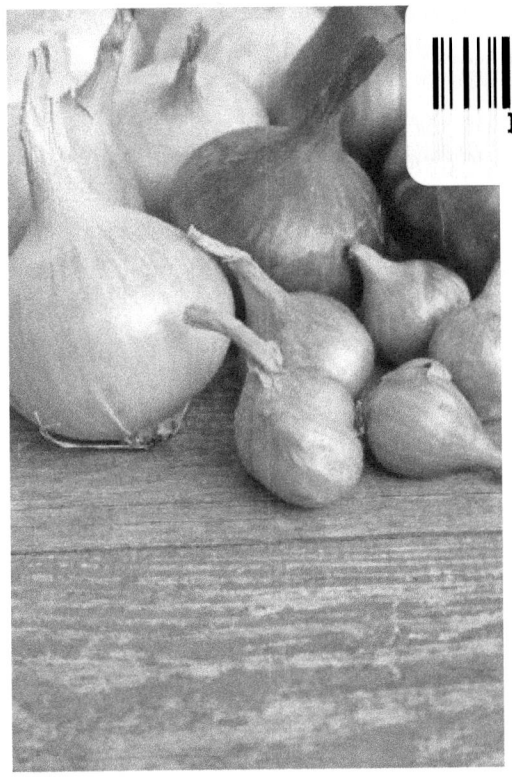

I0421520

Health Learning Series

Dueep Jyot Singh

Mendon Cottage Books

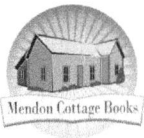

JD-Biz Publishing

Disclaimer

The information is this book is provided for informational purposes only. It is not intended to be used and medical advice or a substitute for proper medical treatment by a qualified health care provider. The information is believed to be accurate as presented based on research by the author.

The contents have not been evaluated by the U.S. Food and Drug Administration or any other Government or Health Organization and the contents in this book are not to be used to treat cure or prevent disease.

The author or publisher is not responsible for the use or safety of any diet, procedure or treatment mentioned in this book. The author or publisher is not responsible for errors or omissions that may exist.

Warning

The Book is for informational purposes only and before taking on any diet, treatment or medical procedure, it is recommended to consult with your primary health care provider.

Our books are available at

1. Amazon.com

2. Barnes and Noble

3. Itunes

4. Kobo

5. Smashwords

6. Google Play Books

Table of Contents

Introduction

I remember an Italian friend, who decided to cook a homemade meal for her hungry family, one leisurely weekend. All the ingredients for a delicious meal were right at hand. Suddenly I heard the song – she sang when she cooked – broken midway and abruptly. Where were the onions? All the herbs were there, and so were the spices. Garlic was also there in large quantities, but where were the onions?

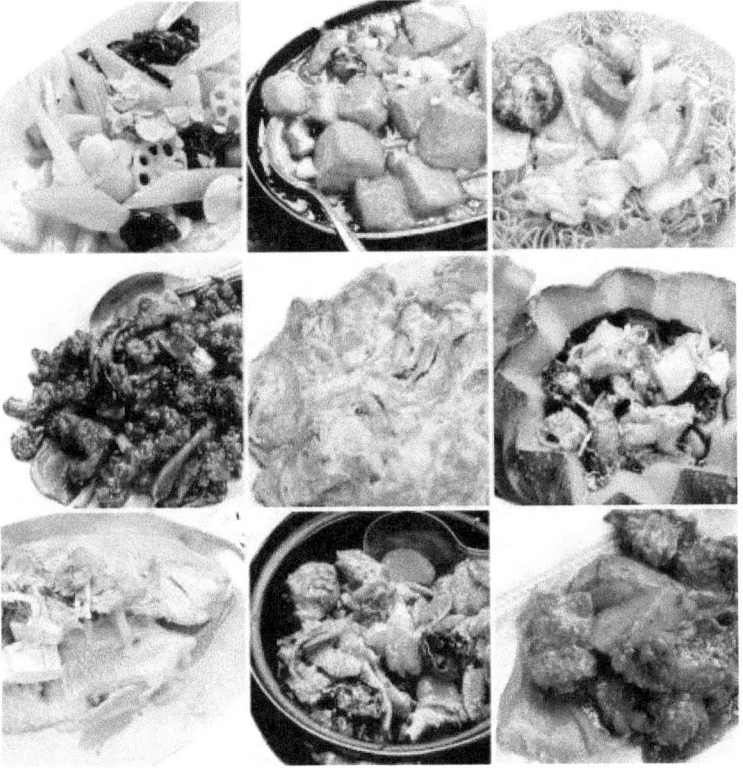

Imagine cuisines from all over the world which have not been flavored with members of the onion family like onions, garlic, leeks, and shallots.

I can just understand how she felt, especially when a large multitude of people all over the world are not going to consider a meal complete, and less it is been accompanied with onions in some form or the other. There are 325 varieties of onions, found all over the world and it has been shown during archaeological surveys and through historical records that onions and mankind go together, just like bacon and eggs, salt-and-pepper and so on.

You can eat onions raw, boiled, baked, cooked or in any way you wish. It is believed that onions supposedly originated in Western Asia, from where they spread all over the earth. Onions are one of the foods spoken of in the Holy Bible.

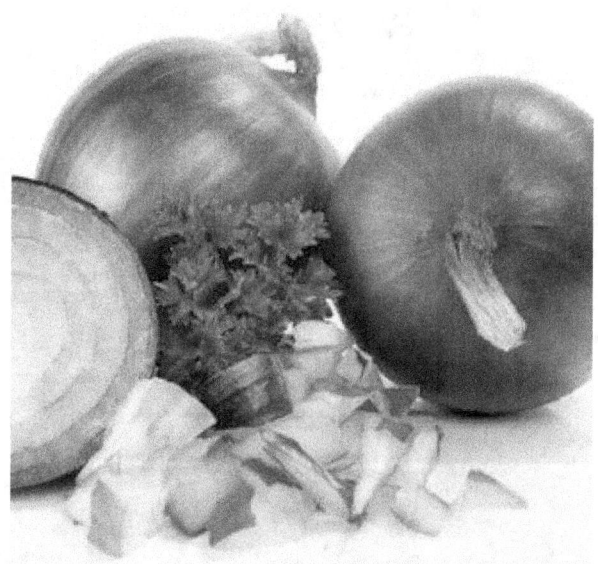

In Egypt, workers on the pyramids were fed corn bread and onions, and so were the soldiers in Rome, who ate bread, onions and a fish sauce called garum, flavored with their daily ration of salt [salarium was the money paid out to them so that they could buy salt.] Thus the term "salary" and the term of loyalty, coming down from the ages, "Eating someone's salt "which means having worked for them. In medieval Europe, rents were paid in onions and also bride gifts given during medieval weddings included onions and spices for those who could afford to give these preferred and desired gifts.

It is a not so well-known fact that the onion is most powerful when it is plucked out fresh from the earth, and eaten within an hour. That is because it has a vital element, which remains only for an hour after the onion has been harvested. So when we were young, our grandmother always told us to go out in the garden and pull out a couple of fresh onion plants, to eat with our lunch.

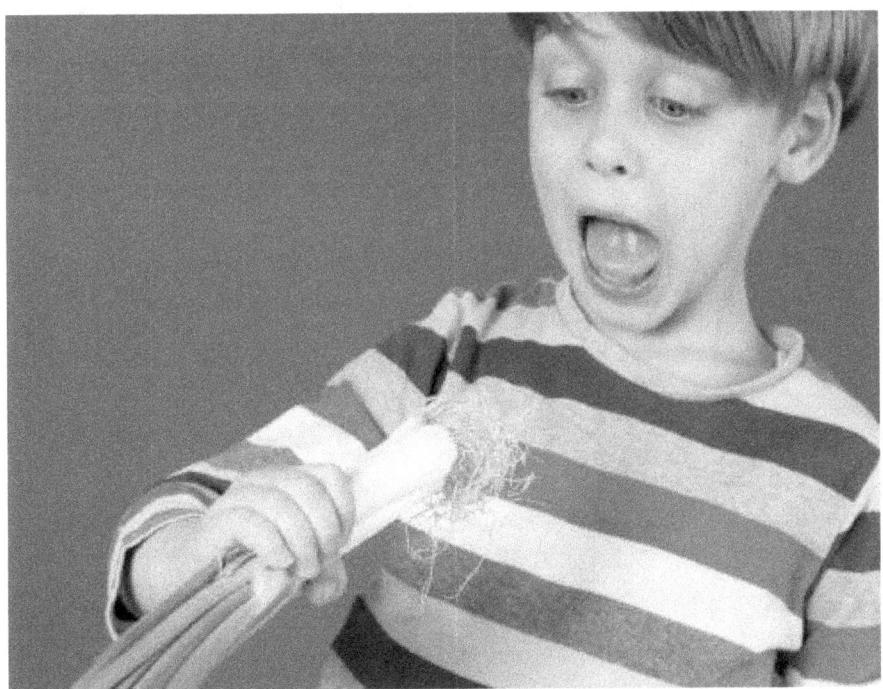

According to her, this would prevent us from suffering from sunstroke. It would also strengthen our immunity systems. It also kept our digestive system working excellently. After lunch, we were made to brush our teeth and gargle with salt water so that we did not go back to school, smelling of onion breath.

It is a known historical fact that Gen. Grant demanded onions from the war Dept. during the American Civil War. According to him, his Army would not keep healthy, without onions, nor would it march without them! The very next morning two wagon loads of onions were sent straight to him.

According to him, onions kept his soldiers fit and prevented them from suffering from stomach problems. He was right, there.

In ancient times, Egyptian priests and aristocrats took their oath of fealty to Pharaoh and country with an onion on their right palm. This can be seen in their wall paintings. According to Nero, it was the regular eating of onions which had cleared up his singing voice and made it sweet and melodious. But that did not prevent the populace and his soldiers, thoroughly bored with his homicidal and maniacal tendencies from slaughtering him wholesale.

Types of Onions

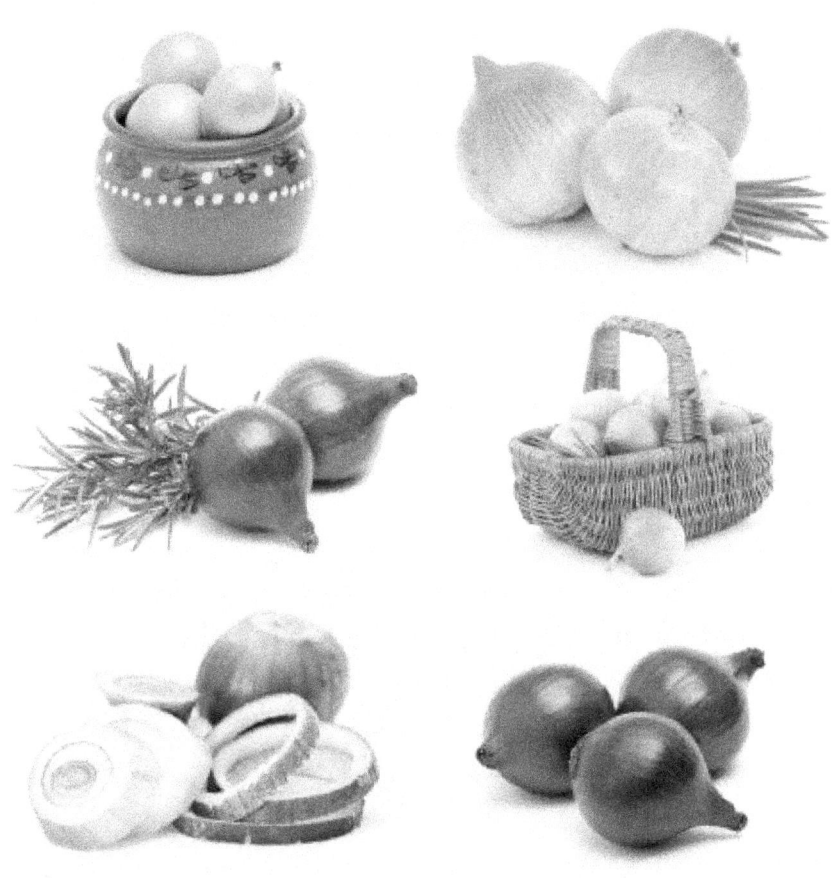

White Onions

Apart from white onions, there are different types of onions available all over the world. You have them in different shapes like round, oval, large in size, small ones, and even flat ones which are used often for pickling purposes. They are considered to be the most superior varieties among the onions.

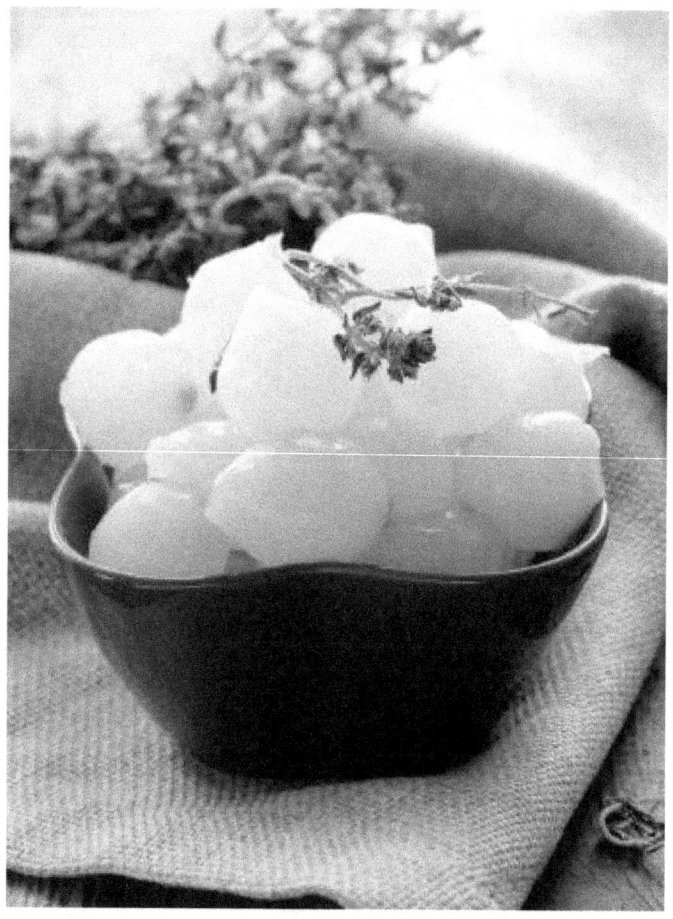

Red onions

This is the most popular variety of onions, found commonly all over the world. These onions are sometimes called the Italian onions. You are going to find the onion layers underneath the skin to be somewhat light blue-ish red in color. They are excellent for salads.

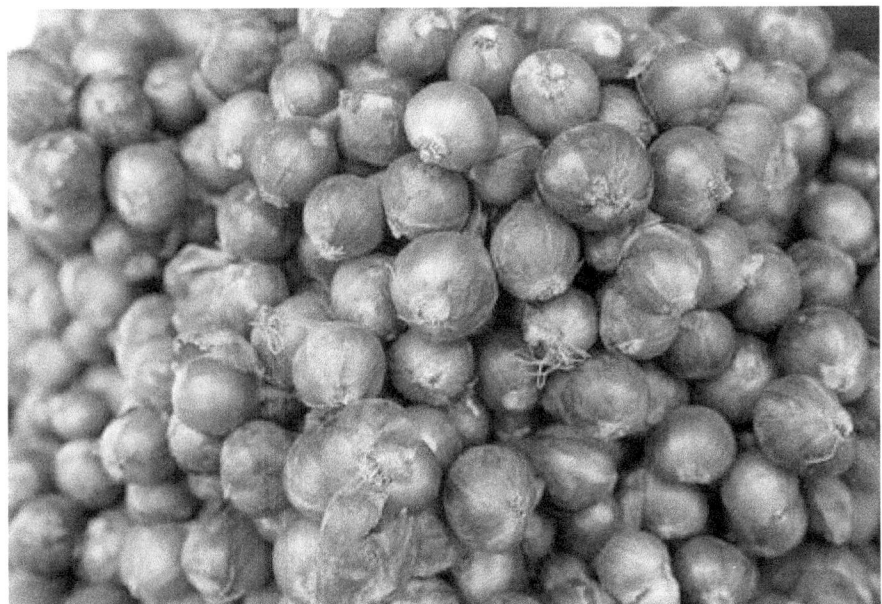

Pink/Yellow Onions

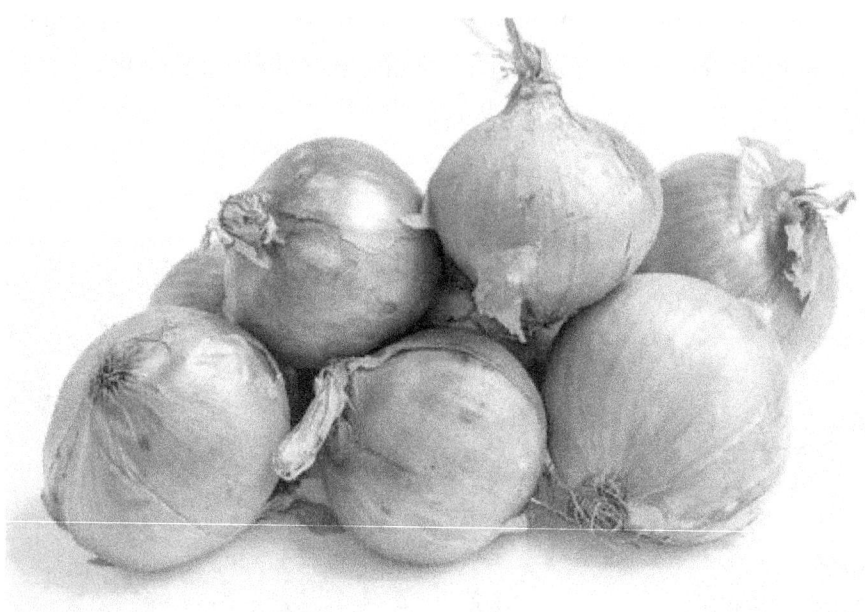

These are also onion varieties, which are very commonly available in the markets. You are either going to find them hanging in bunches or they are going to be piled up to be added to your marketing basket.

Leafy Onions

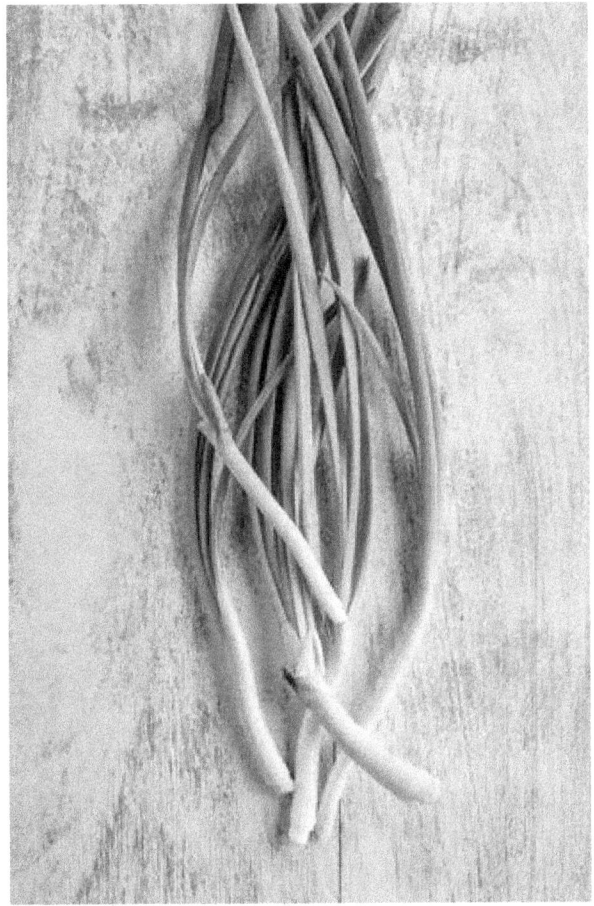

These are the onions, which are green, and which have been freshly harvested from your garden, before they have had time to mature. What I remember best about these leafy onions, when plucked from our garden was breaking off two inch pieces of the "leaves", and "whistling" through them.

Children down the ages have instinctively found that these onion leaves are excellent musical instruments, just with a little bit of creativity and experimentation![1]

These leaves, along with the chopped up portions of the young onions were excellent in soups and potages. They were also eaten raw in salads. Also, they were excellent filling material along with mashed potatoes to stuff pancakes and breads. Apart from that, they have always been an excellent addition to omelet's, stir fry dishes, and also in mayonnaise/bread spread along with other herbs.

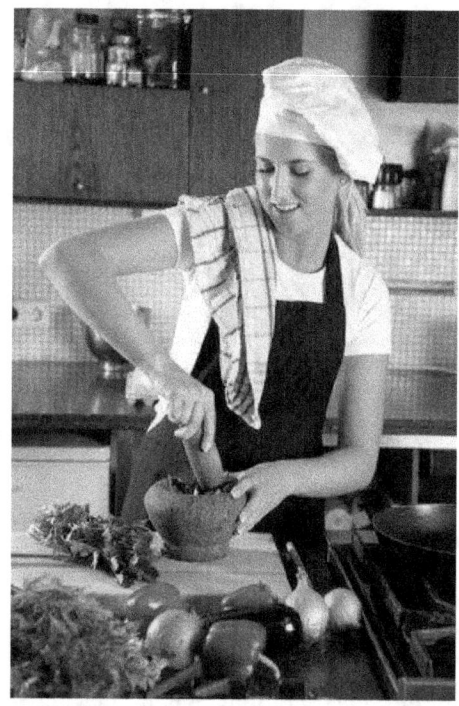

---

[1] Same thing with Combs wrapped up in paper...

These particular leafy and immature onions are preferred by people who do not like the strong flavor, taste and aroma of mature onions. That is why they eat them fried, ground, boiled and mixed with other vegetables to add flavor and texture to a meal, which would otherwise have been unappetizing and bland.

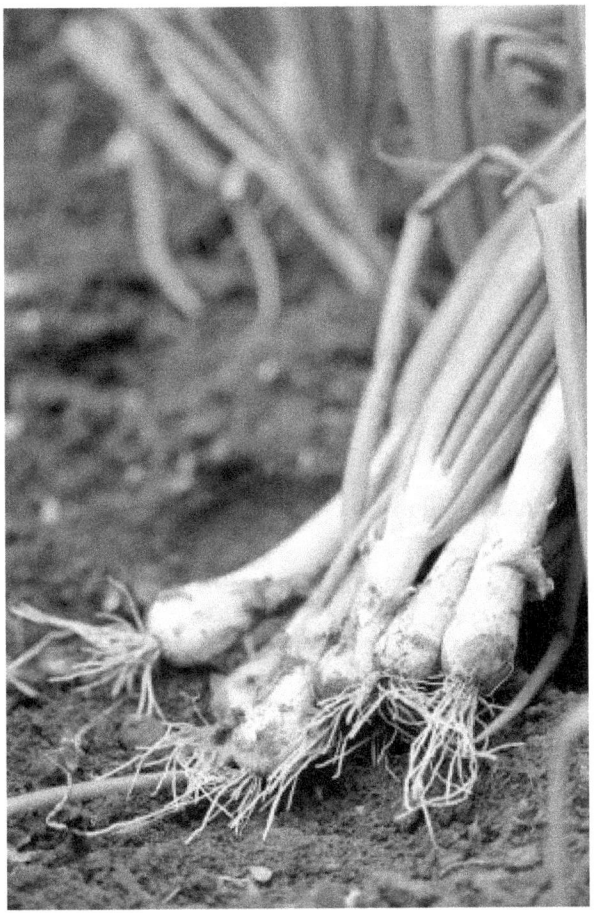

Down the ages, people have been using mediums like salt, vinegar and honey to lessen and counteract the powerful effects of onions. If you find them very strong, you can try dipping them in salt water for a while. I do that to counteract the sulfur content in the onions, before I chop them up. No tears, no fears!

Onions are perennial herbs and their bulbs are going to vary in size, shape, color and onions. You can get them in cultivar form or in their native form. The color ranges going to be anywhere from white to yellow and green to red. The shape is going to be flat, spherical or spear shaped.

Italian and Bermuda onions are flat and large they are known to be fairly mild in taste Spanish varieties, sweet, juicy and large. The scientific name of onion is *Allium Cepa* and it belongs to the Liliaceae family.

Leading world producers of onions include China, USA, India, Japan, Russia, and Turkey. The most popular common names by which they are recognized all over the world is loyon, white globe onion, oignon, red globe onion, and the Spanish onion.

Onions contain 86% water, 11.6% carbohydrates, 1.2% protein, .7% fat, .18% calcium .7% iron, and .5% phosphorus.

Onions for Nutrition

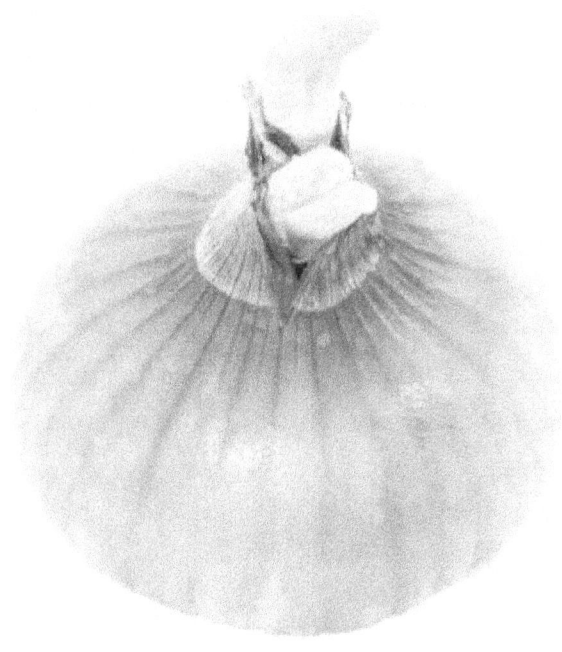

Apart from the culinary usage of onions, many people in the West are beginning to understand the power of herbs as medicines. The annual sale of medicinal herbs the USA alone is more than $2 billion! According to the WHO, more than 80% of the people in the world rely on traditional form of health care. The onion is said to be the oldest cultivated herb, and that is why even ancient Greek, Egyptian, Chinese, Japanese, Korean etc. medical treatises speak about onion remedies in order to cure ailments.

However, it is surprising to see that ancient Indian alternative medicine remedies, especially homeopathic medicines asked the patients not to eat onions, while the treatment was being done. According to an ancient Chinese traveler, I Tsing traveling in the Indian subcontinent more than 900 years ago, Indians believed that eating onions of any kind caused poor eyesight and weaken the body and also caused progressive degeneration. This was centuries ago. Fortunately, better sense prevailed, and Indians soon found out that this idea was nonsense. And now, nearly every cuisine in nearly every region in this continent uses onions in the composition of good and healthy food. That is because about 600 years ago, during the Mogul invasion of India, a new cuisine and a new medicinal science was brought to India from Central Asia. Thereafter, the onion became irreplaceable in the kitchen as well as in the medical cabinet.

By the mid-19th century, the onion was a favorable pot vegetable of people who had once shunned it, and no curry could do without it.

According to the ancient Egyptians, this spherical bulb was a symbol of the universe and they believed that the onions kept Evil spirits away. The evil spirits, I suppose were kept away with the pungent odor of sulfur. When the onion bulb is crushed, sulfoxides are released.

The pungent odor is due to the thiosulfate content present in the onion. The active antiallergic and anti-inflammatory ingredients of the onion are flavonoids, which are capable of releasing histamine. This is the mediator of inflammation. Onions also contain an immune system boosting element – selenium.

They say an apple a day keeps the doctor away, but onions are equally effective. In traditional medicine, are considered to be a cure for almost every conceivable illness under the sun. One may think that to be an exaggeration, but ancient medical treatises have lots of remedies using onions and onion juice to cure diseases ranging from baldness to constipation.

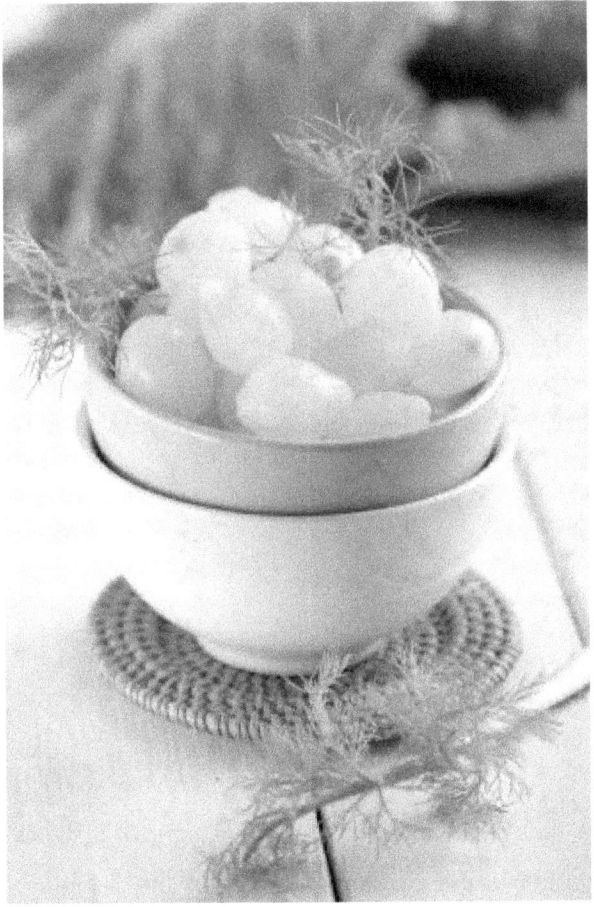

That is because the sulfur compounds made the onions antiseptic and antibacterial. In ancient Chinese medicine onions were used to cure colds, ear aches, laryngitis, animal bites, warts and even gunpowder burns. They were also used to get rid of parasites in the stomach as well as a rejuvenating tonic.

Onions for Diabetics

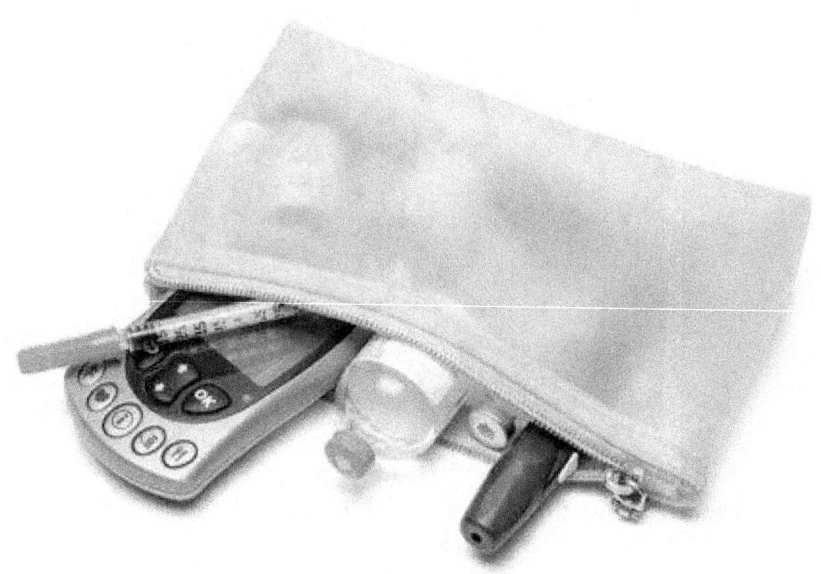

Diabetes can be controlled by onions.

Diabetes is as old as mankind, but now an epidemic of diabetes is sweeping all over the world because of changing lifestyles and changing food habits. The number of 150 million patients with diabetes in the world in 2000 has nearly doubled to 275 million patients today and growing. Diabetes occurs when the pancreas, the second-largest gland fails to regulate the glucose concentration of the blood.

If the blood sugar is uncontrolled, it is going to damage all the organs of the body leading to diabetic coma and death.

According to herbalists, the cure and treatment for diabetes, lies in your kitchen and has been in use for centuries. You just need to increase your intake of raw onions. They possess blood sugar lowering properties and have been used since ancient times, along with bitter gourd to help contain and cure diabetes.

Try a mixture of the juice of one onion and one bitter gourd[2] every day for about seven days, first thing in the morning, and then check your blood sugar levels. You are going to be surprised at the improvement.

---

[2] Here is a bitter gourd juice episode in the interesting life and times of yours truly. About a decade ago, I was working with a company, where colleagues and faculty members had lunch together, along with our boss, every lunch time. His wife prepared fresh bitter gourd juice for him, and sent it by the hand of their servant in a huge thermos flask. This was how his diabetes was being kept under control.

New faculty members were accepted as part of the team only when the boss invited them to toss off a glass of that delicious looking sparkling light green juice. Naturally, he hated the bitter juice, and all the other colleagues managed to keep poker faces when the newcomer was asked to drink up that healthy drink. Lighthearted hazing office style!

So here was I with this brimming glass in front of me and with everybody trying not to look interested in the proceedings. I tossed it off, licked my chops and said "hmmm, good, what is it?" In answer, the boss immediately handed me his thermos full of the juice and said, "if you like it, you can drink it" in, no pun intended, bitter tones, while the rest of the table split its sides! He knew what would happen next. The servant would go home and report to his mistress that Sir had given the glass to the new manager, and she had said that it was very nice! That means he would never have any excuse not to drink his daily quota of bitter gourd juice.

Needless to say, his diabetes condition is under control, and has not been aggravated any more. Also, that is because along with the bitter gourd, he had to eat plenty of raw onions, freshly plucked from the garden, and sent to the office lunchroom.

Onions for Stomach Problems

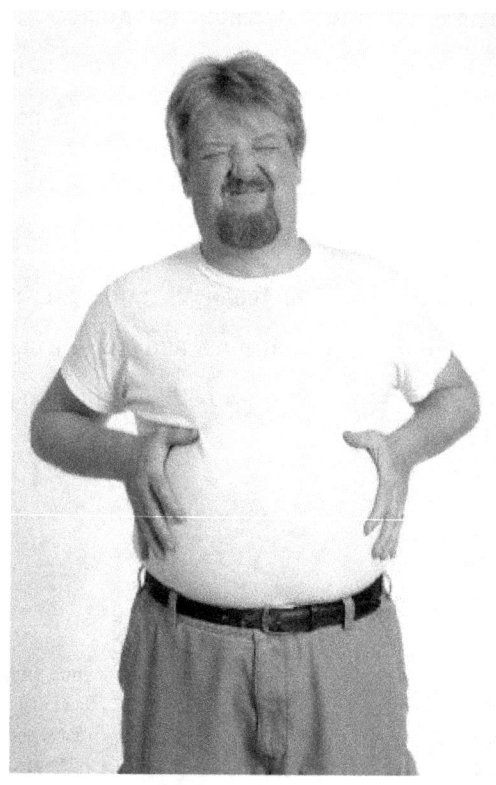

Onions are excellent digesters, anti-flatulent, and anti-inflammatory and therefore they are going to keep stomach ache, abdominal discomfort and bloating at bay. According to Dutch researchers, people consuming a large amount of onions have 50% less chance of suffering from any sort of gastrointestinal cancer. In the same way, it has been proven that a healthy serving of a combination of scallions, onion and garlic in your daily meal is going to provide you from the development of prostate cancer.

Using onions for curing mild stomach ailments like Tummy aches and bloating can be done very easily. The traditional way is to take one teaspoonful of onion juice, add a pinch of rock salt, and one pinch of asafoetida,[3] which is a traditional powerful spice. This simple traditional medicinal recipe is going to have an amazing effect on your digestive system. Not only is it going to cure rate from any sort of problem, but it is going to strengthen it.

---

[3] There is some interesting information about this particular spice, on this URL – http://en.wikipedia.org/wiki/Asafoetida

Diarrhea and Cholera Preventative

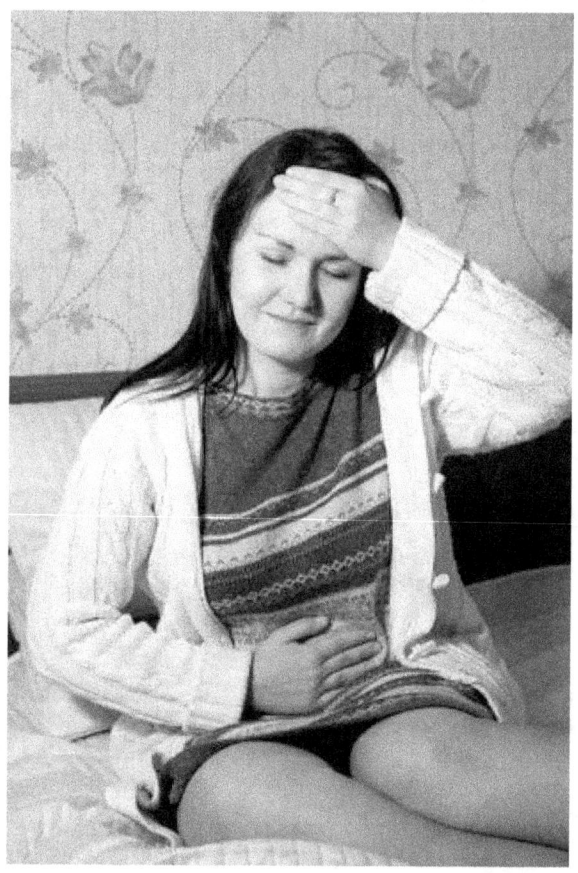

If you are suffering from constipation, all you have to do is consume raw onions with your meals. The antibacterial and antifungal properties of onions were long known to control food poisoning. That is why in medieval times, when they did not bother about cooking and eating rotten meat, no wonder they ate onions and garlic in large quantities and thus managed to survive salmonella poisoning.

In many parts of the East, where cholera and diarrhea happens to be a regular endemic every summer, infections and stomach problems were prevented with the consumption of lots of raw onions.

It is a well-known fact that the British had a tough time in India, especially in the summers while they ruled the Indian subcontinent. They died like flies due to cholera, every summer. That was because they considered the alternative traditional medicines to be savage and barbaric and would never listen to reason. Apart from that, they did not eat raw onions, because according to them, that was something eaten by Italians and the French, the latter who were their traditional enemies.

So onion eaters and garlic eaters were looked down upon by the sensitive-nosed British. They could not bear the aroma of sulfur fumes. Also, according to them, onions were something eaten by the natives, and definitely not by the Superior Race. They had the same attitude, even when they were in Africa, especially Egypt. And that is why they did not have a good immunity system working for them, when the rains came. And so they perished and blamed it all on the hot climate.

Onions to prevent Cholesterol buildup

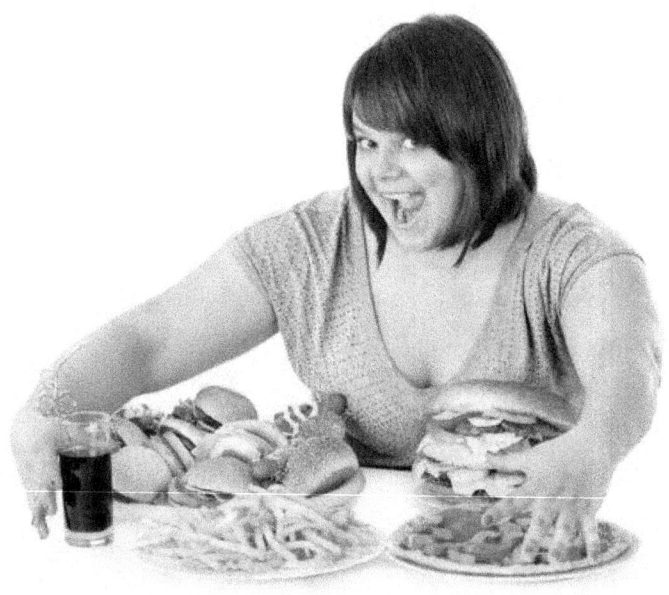

Many people are under the impression that cholesterol is the only factor which causes heart attacks. That is not true. Cholesterol, which is a fat like substance that we get from two sources – the food we eat, and which is manufactured by our liver is one of the factors which contributes to heart ailments.

Your liver is going to place cholesterol into packages called lipoproteins. These are made up of lipids and proteins. These lipoproteins are of three types – VLDL – very low density lipoprotein, LDL – low-density lipoprotein and HDL – high density lipoprotein.

Out of these the low-density lipoprotein is bad cholesterol because it is going to stick easily along the walls of the blood vessels in your body. It has been revealed by a number of studies that onions are anticholesterolaemic and reduce the chances of cholesterol buildup in your system.

That is because onions maintain a contain watch over LDL. They do not allow it to block the blood vessels. Onions also have other heart friendly benefits. They are natural anticlotting agents. That means you are not going to suffer from blood clots, in your system, if you eat lots of onions. That is because this consumption of onions is going to keep the blood thin and flowing properly through your circulatory system

Also, onions are capable of increasing fibrinolysin, which is going to suppress the platelet aggregation associated with a high-fat diet. This fibrinolysin is also capable of retarding the age dependent changes in your blood vessels. These actions are going to keep your heart healthy and pumping.

Onions for Urinary Infections

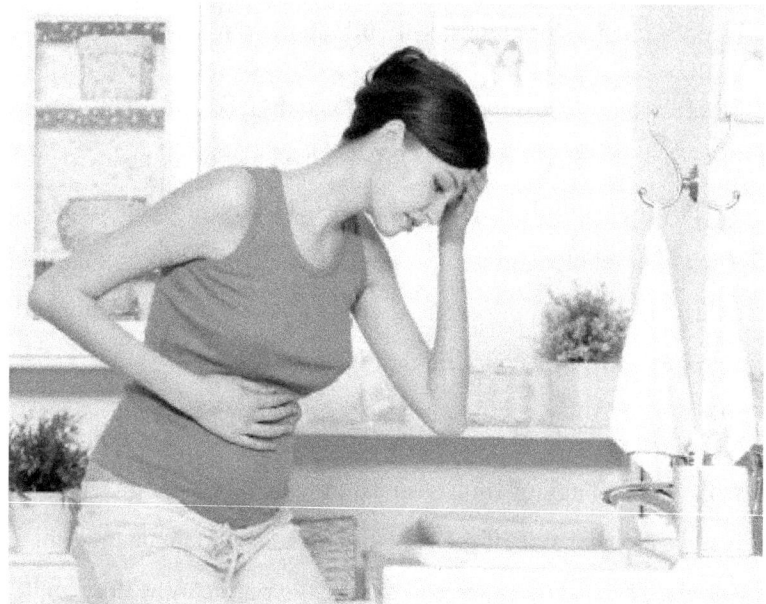

Toxic waste products are capable of accumulating in the urine. These materials accumulated provide favorable conditions for the growth of microbes in your urinary tract. Women are more prone to urinary infections because of their biological and physical makeup.

Onions are diuretics, which are going to flush out the waste products and the germs, during the elimination process from the body. They also control the inflammation of the bladder. Antibacterial properties of onions will also make sure that you do not suffer from any inflammation or infection caused by toxic wastes.

Inflammation of Joints and Osteoarthritis

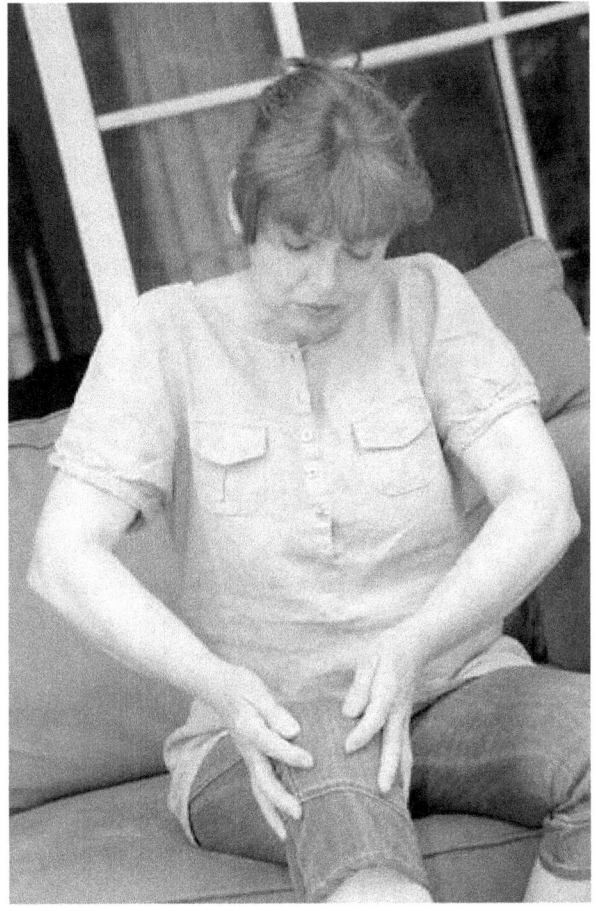

One of the common waste products produced by the body is uric acid. It normally passes out through the kidneys. But sometimes, there is more production of uric acid, formed in the body than which has been eliminated. These are now going to settle in your body has uric acid crystals.

When these crystals are caught in the spaces between joints the tissue surrounding those affected joints become inflamed. These inflamed joints irritate the nerve endings that supply the joint producing a lot of pain. This is what happens in gout.

Another common disease of the joints is osteoarthritis. It is going to develop when the cartilage around the joints, especially of is and the hips wears away with the passage of time. New bone tissue growing beneath prevents the joints from moving as smoothly as they should, naturally.

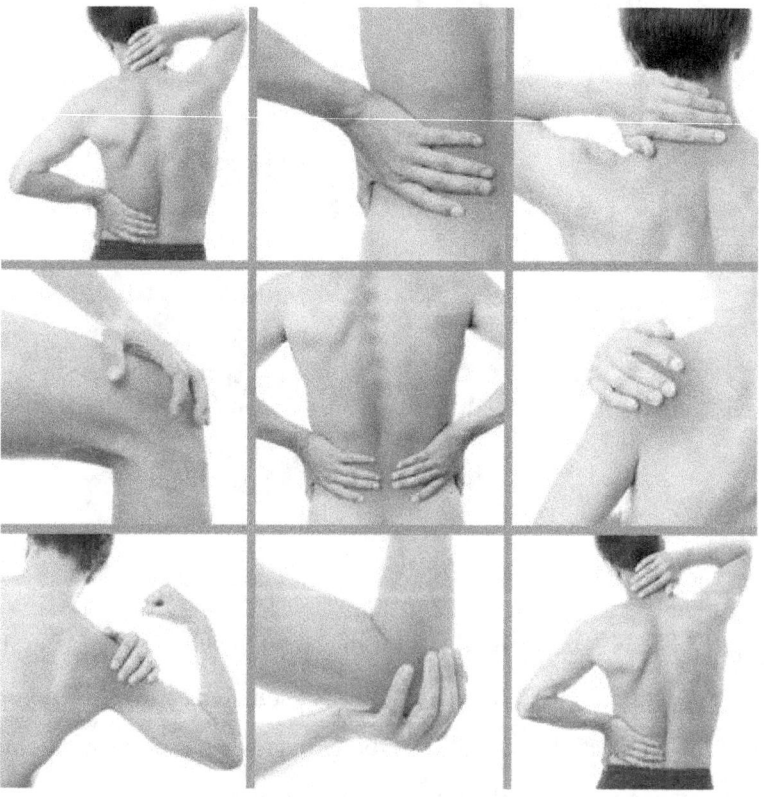

Onions have been traditionally used to get rid of painful joints and alleviate the pain. For this you need to mix equal quantities of onion juice and warm mustard oil. Apply this mixture on the affected joints. And then sit back and watch the miraculous results.

Mustard oil is very strong and very pungent. That is why, you will need to do this massage at a time, and in an area where and when you are not disturbed by people who may appear and say, "Golly, what a pong!"

Why am I talking about mustard oil? Why did I not say coconut oil, or olive oil or any other softer, sweeter smelling oil? That is because mustard oil, like I said is very powerful. It also has extremely strong and beneficial immediate healing quantities.

Surprisingly enough, this strong oil has never been used to heal people in many parts of the West, because they do not like the strong aroma of this thick and viscous oil.

Onions to Cure Depression

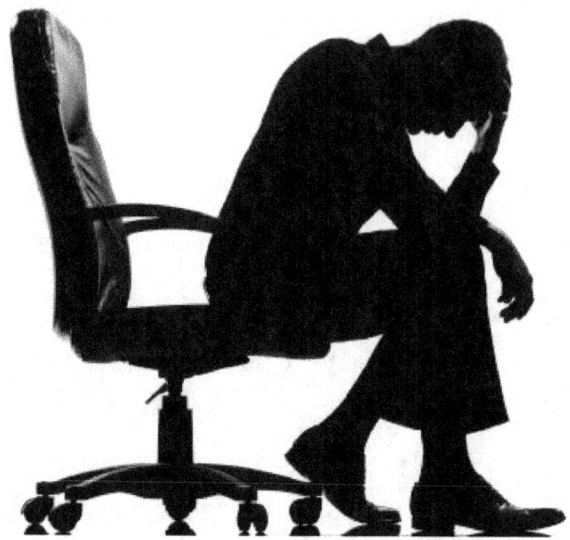

It has been scientifically proven that people who do not have enough of selenium in their meals are more prone to nervous fatigue, depression and anxiety. I guess that is why aristocratic females in Europe, especially Britain, spent so much of their time fainting away daintily, because their nerves were so sensitive and tender! In fact, lots of "delicately" brought up women in the Regency era and in the 19th century cultivated this affectation and resorting to Sal volatile at the drop of a straw bonnet.

I would call that affectation and ennui working overtime, just because they did not have anything constructive to do. More onions in their diet and more physical labor outdoors and they would have forgotten everything about megrims, depression, hysteria, fainting spells, nervous problems and even supposed nervous fatigue – all of which they cultivated in order to show people all around them, how refined they were.

If you happen to belong to that category, try adding onions, garlic and leeks to your diet. Your ancestors and their neighbors definitely did not have any problem eating these healthy foods for centuries. How did you become such a languishing and affected lily with your possibly ridiculous airs and graces?

The selenium in balance in your family is going to set your moods and possible depression on the right path to health.

Onions to cure Coughs and Colds

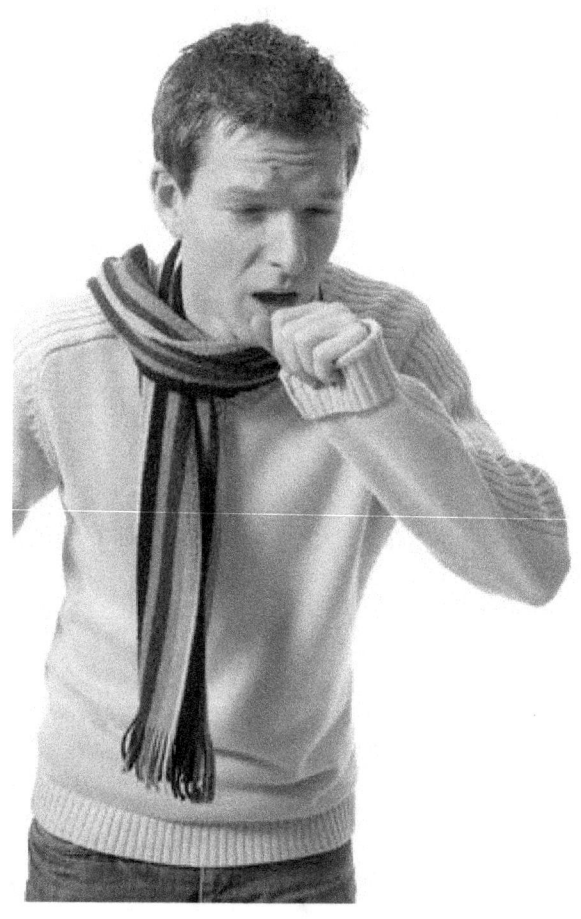

Here comes the winter season, and viruses are going to infect your throat, nose, lungs, and larynx. Most of us spend a lot of our winter time suffering from influenza and from cough and cold, which could have easily been prevented by just the addition of more onions in our diet. Just take onion juice and honey mixed in equal amounts, three – four times a day, and never suffer from any of these infections again.

This magic mixture is powerful enough as a natural expectorant. It is going to calm down your cough. You can also find it very useful in attacks of breathlessness, especially in asthma. Along with this, there is an unexpected side benefit – the onion and honey mixture is capable of getting rid of that extra weight and poundage in your body. Try it out!

Anti-aging benefits Of Onions

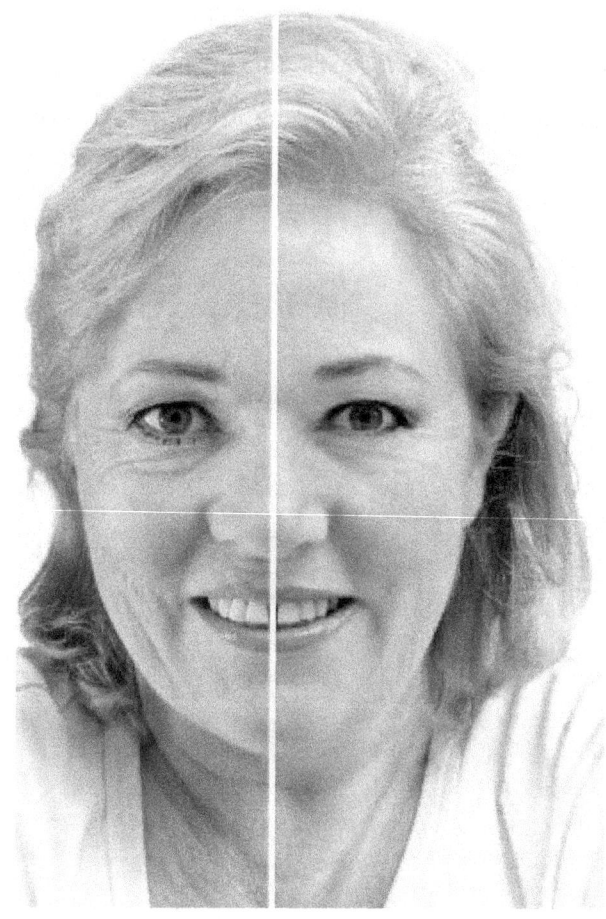

If I had been born 500 years ago, in a place where I did not have to bother about disease and destruction through war, I would have lived a long life, with plenty of youthful looks, even with the passing of time. That was because I would have access to plenty of fresh air, opportunities to do lots of exercise outdoors and eat plenty of fruits and vegetables which did not have access to chemical fertilizers and poisoned air and soil.

However, thanks to the strides science has made in the 21st century, there are very few pockets of untouched water and air left on the surface of the earth. Free radicals are caused by stress, pollution, smoking and fried food. The changing lifestyle is also going to have a disastrous effect on your health. The free radicals are going to attack, alter and destroy your normal cells. These lead to degenerative illnesses like strokes, hypertension and cancer.

These free radicals also interfere with collagen synthesis. This is going to result in wrinkles and sagging of the skin. Onions, which are rich in flavonoids, are going to fight these rogue elements and molecules. They are also going to restore the disease busting tools provided to us by nature. This means that the more onions you eat, the more you are going to protect yourself against aging symptoms.

Onion Juice to Remove Scars

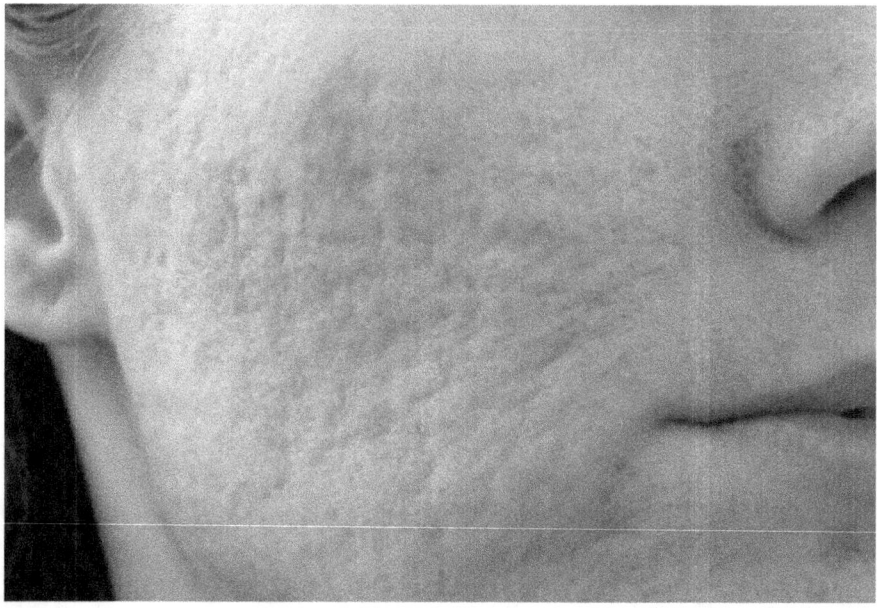

This is something which I saw being used in a remote village somewhere up in the mountains. Onion juice was spread over wounds and scars in order to remove the marks and heal the wounds.

I would like you to try this experiment out for yourself. Choose a scar on your body, which you want to remove. Mix equal quantities of onion juice and honey with half a teaspoonful of turmeric powder. Remember turmeric powder stains the skin, so you will have to remove that dried paste from your skin, 20 minutes later with a spoonful of yogurt. This time is to allow the onion juice and the honey to get absorbed in the skin.

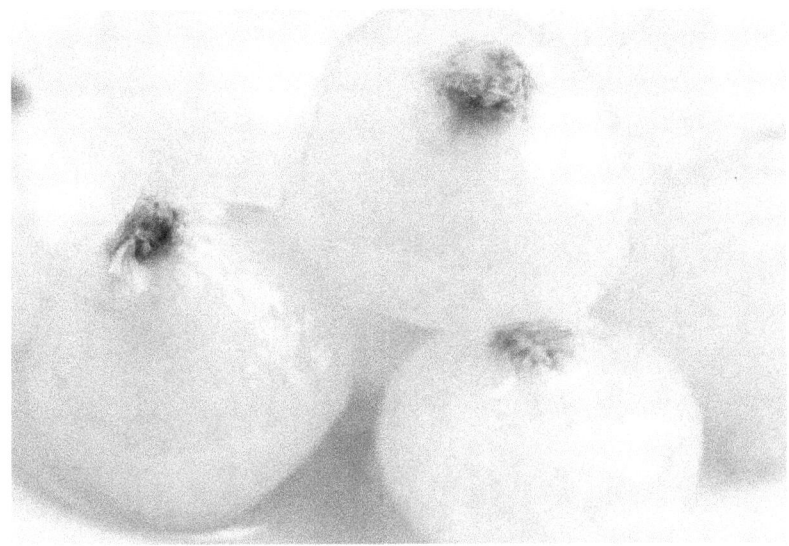

Try this out for about one week. You are going to see fresh cells growing in the scar area and the diminishing of that injured portion. I used this recipe to get rid of a scar burn on my hand. Incidentally, there happened to be a small wart growing near the scar, and it also disappeared when I dabbed it with the onion juice and honey mix.

Onions for Sunstroke

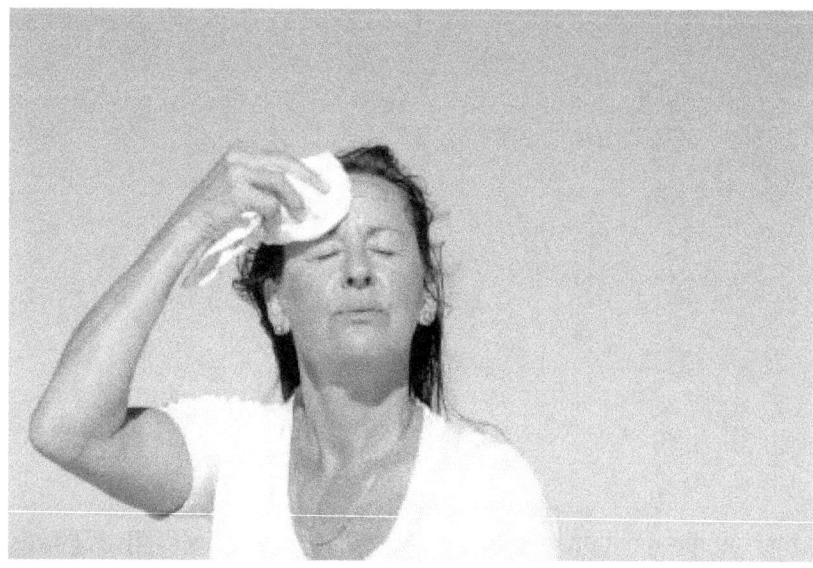

Prolonged exposure to the sun is going to upset the body's heat regulating mechanism that means the body temperature is going to rise from the normal value of 98°F to 104°F or higher. A person under such circumstances is going to feel flushed, have a heightened temperature and a strong rapid pulse.

I remember one terrible summer about two decades ago, when I was traveling on a hot summer afternoon, visiting some family members in the city. The temperature was 111°F in the afternoon. I got onto the bus, in the state of half delirious sunstroke, without even knowing it, got off at the bus stop, and staggered home totally incoherent and like a walking zombie. Incidentally, my temperature was 104.2°F, to the great horror of my father!

Anybody else would have just collapsed and expired but I staggered into the bathroom in that state of delirium and put my head under a shower, while the rest of the family kept looking at me astonished, wondering if I was inebriated in the afternoon.

After that, I collapsed on the bed and went off into a deep sleep, for about six hours which restored me.

When I woke up I was given onion juice and buttermilk to get rid of the aftereffects of the sunstroke which luckily had not managed to curdle my brains – according to the rest of the relatives – and this is what happened to dim bulbs, who went out in the sun without proper headgear, sun protection in the shape of umbrellas, and drinking lots of water before they ventured out in the midday sun.

If my grandmother would have been alive then, she would have rubbed raw onions on my temples, stomach, soles of my feet and palms. That was the ancient traditional way of getting rid of the aftereffects of sun stroke.

Remember overexposure to the sun is potentially lethal. So do not go out in the afternoon sun, unless absolutely necessary.

Onions as an Appetite Enhancer

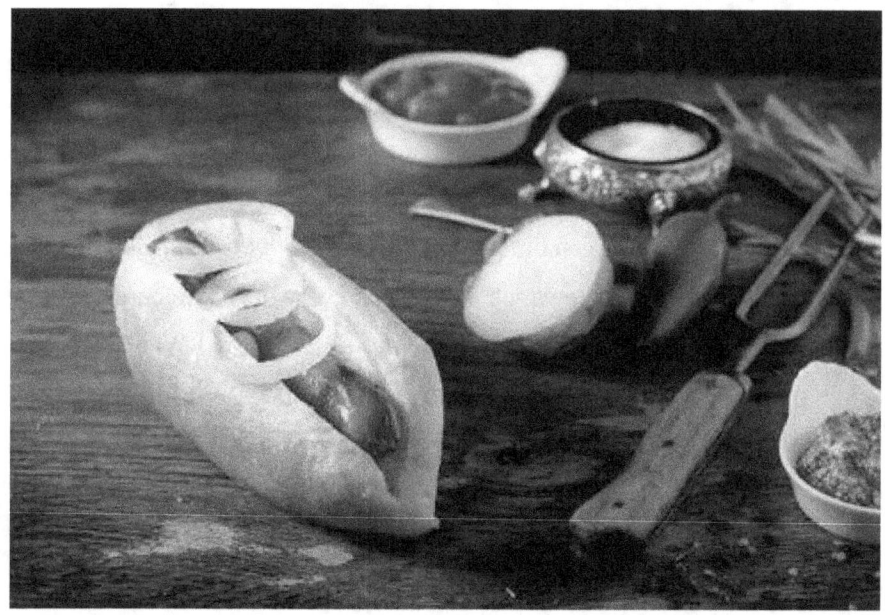

Try out this experiment when you do not want to eat anything. Unfortunately, many of us are suffering from eating disorders because we wish to lose weight, or we have just stopped eating because we are too busy to do so. And this is going to have a detrimental effect on our appetites and thus on our health. That is why most of us pretend that we are not hungry, and we soon reach a stage when we stop feeling hungry because we have conditioned our minds to ignore the pains of hunger.

This is an extremely harmful trend and if you belong to that section of misguided mankind, just order a dish which has a number of onions in it and smell it. The aroma of onions is an appetite enhancer. It is going to give your dull appetite a wake-up call.

That is why good cooks are liberal when using onions in sandwiches, hamburgers, soups and salads. Apart from a good-looking garnish, these onions are going to add flavor, taste, and texture to your meals.

I once saw a kid in a burger joint removing all the onions from his burger, because he did not like the taste. His kid sister immediately grabbed all the onions, calling him a 100% Dumbo,[4] all the while. That made him rather indignant, because there must be something special in the onions which he was not eating and which was so well appreciated by his tiresome nuisance of a kid sister.

So in a state of amusement, I noticed him, tentatively taking a huge bite of his burger without removing the onions. And then suddenly I saw the look of enlightenment on his face. Much as he hated to admit it, his sister had the right of it.

Alas, for all those burgers from which he had removed the onions beforehand! But at least he was lucky that he had found out the difference in taste, a couple of onion rings made to his jumbo burger.

This "kid" is now 32 years old, with 2 children of his own, an excellent gourmet cook, and a super fan of onions in any shape, form, and size. And he is the first one to any salad bowl, grabbing all the onions as and when he can.[5]

---

[4] This supercilious particular tone can only be used by a kid sister/brother and is very irritating-*Duhhhh- mboh!*

[5] His wife leaves the fiddling about in the kitchen to him! Sensible woman. All she has to do is say in a very sincere and appreciative tone, "my, my, what a wonderful

Traditional Onion Recipes

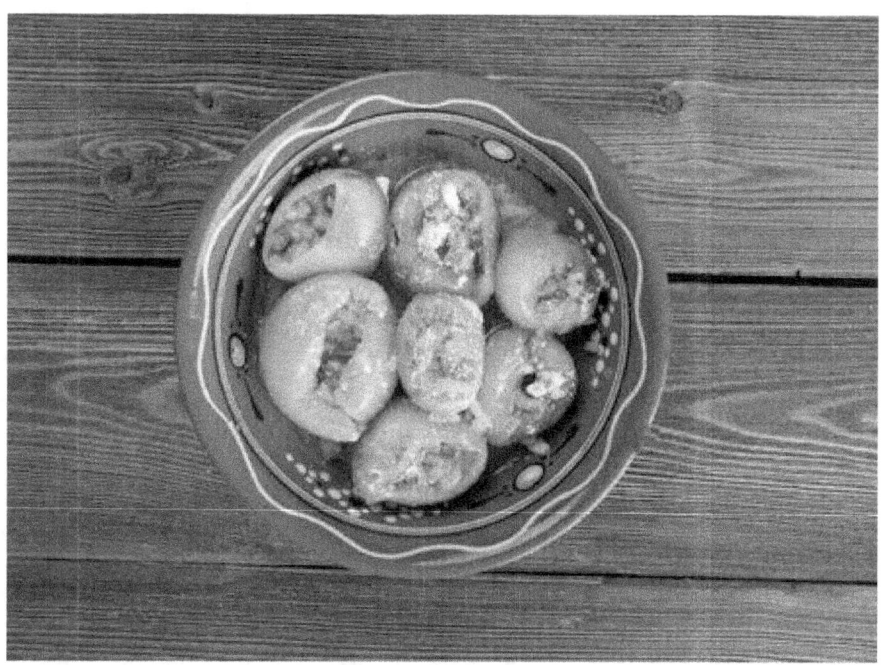

Stuffed Onions

- 10 peeled onions

- 1 bell pepper

- 1 tomato

- 1/4 Tbsp turmeric powder

- 1 Tbsp of oil

---

cook you are, miles better than I am, anytime" and he happily takes on all the kitchen duties. Talk about human psychology.

- hefty pinches of all the available herbs and spices in your cupboards: including parsley, cumin seeds, paprika, pepper, sage, thyme, marjoram, etc.

Trim the top and the bottom of the onions keeping the nodes intact. Make vertical slits from top to the bottom, taking care not to split the onions. Mix all the dry and herbs spices and stuff them into the slits.

Heat the oil and add the cumin seeds. When they are spluttering – this happens when they have been fried a light golden brown – add the chopped up tomato and capsicum. Add the stuffed onions to this frying mixture and also add more spices and herbs, if you want

Add half a cup of water and cook covered until the onions are tender. Serve hot.

Traditional Onion Soup

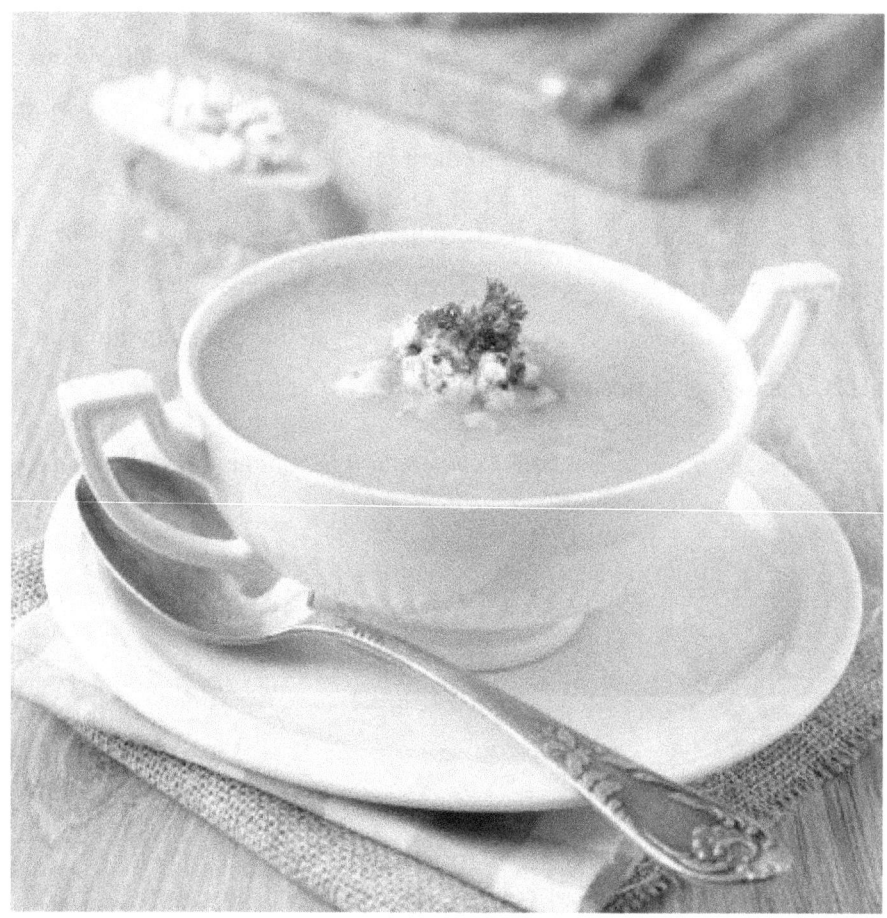

This is a traditional French recipe. More than 500 years ago, Onions and potatoes were popularized among the populace by the then King, who used human psychology. His head botanist Parmentier sowed potatoes in a field, and when they were ready to harvest, the field was guarded with a unit of soldiers.

Naturally, the populace wanted to know what was so precious, which needed to be guarded so carefully. But the soldiers accidentally-on-purpose were careless in their sentry duty, and within one night, the whole field was harvested by the citizens of France, who stole away into the darkness with those tubers called potatoes.

And now potatoes are an integral part of French cuisine. In the same manner onions were popularized by the aristocracy given permission to wear onion flowers in their coat labels as boutonnieres. Once the populace saw them doing that, everyone wanted to grow onions for those delicate onion flowers. And so onions became an important part of French cuisine.

Time needed for preparation of this traditional onion soup is 25 minutes. Cooking time is 20 minutes and this soup is enough for four hungry people.

- **4 large onions**

- **3 Tbsp butter**

- **1 Tbsp of olive oil**

- **1 Tbsp of flour**

- **1/2 cup of white wine**

- **4 cups of water**

- **Salt and pepper, to taste**

- **1/2 cup of grated cheese**

- **6 slices of sandwich bread**

Peel and mince the onions. Mix them up in the butter and the oil.

Mix the flour with warm water, the white wine and season with salt-and-pepper, according to taste.

Bring the flour – water mixture and the onion mixture to a boil, covered and cooked at low heat for 20 minutes.

Grill the bread sandwiches and make some of them into bread crumbs. Place them at the bottom of your soup bowls and powder with grated cheese. Pour the hot onion soup over this bread and cheese.

Powder the rest of the cheese and some bread crumbs on top of the soup. You may want to place them under the grill for some time in order to melt the cheese on top. Serve piping hot.

How to Dry Onions

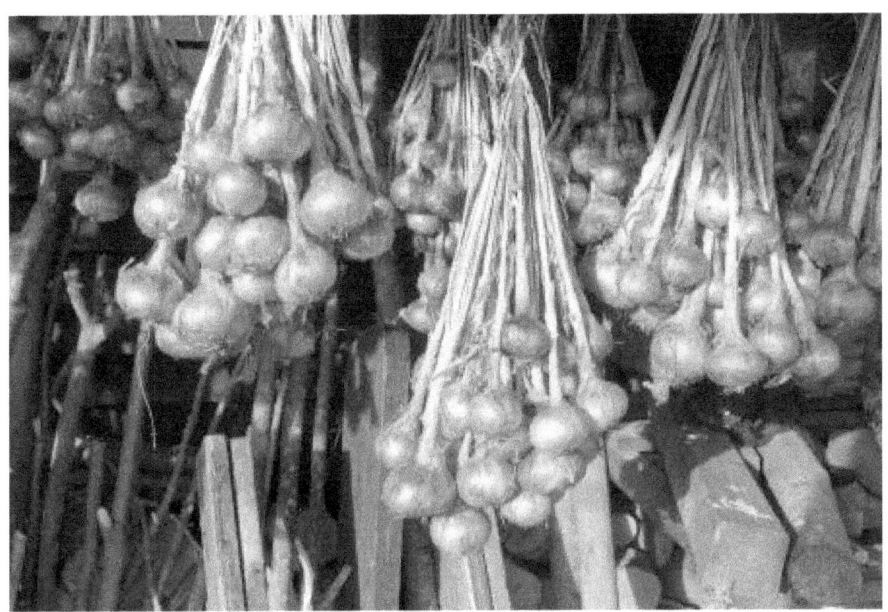

Onion powder is extremely easy to make. Just collect your onions and chop them into small pieces, and dry them in the sun [in a shady place] for four – five days, till the onions shrivel up. Naturally, I did this in summer. Then grind this dried onion in your mixer, and sieve. After that, sun dry it for another half an hour before bottling in a glass bottle.

You can also dry these pieces in your oven at the lowest temperature or in your desiccator/dehydrator.

Conclusion

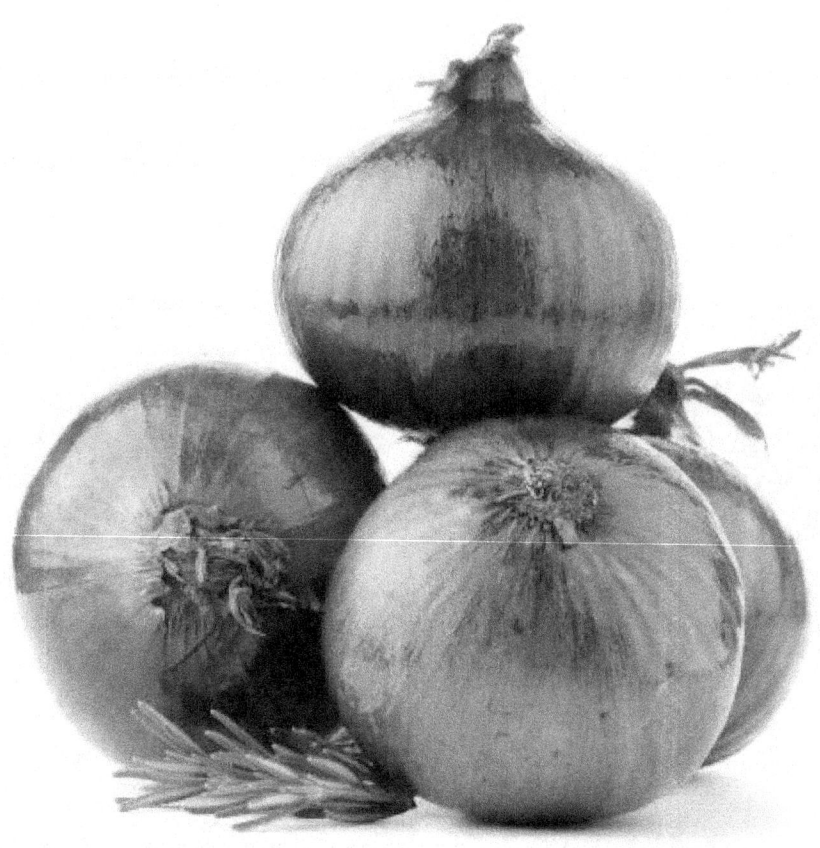

This book gives you plenty of information about onions and how you can keep healthy with them. These herbs have been an integral part of human life for millenniums.

You can get more information on onions and how to grow them in these books published by us.

The Magic of Onions:

http://www.amazon.com/Magic-Onions-Cuisine-Health-Learning-ebook/dp/B00HYLZ6U2/ref=sr_1_5?ie=UTF8&qid=1440029963&sr=8-5&keywords=the+magic+of+onions

Introduction to the Onion Family:

http://www.amazon.com/Introduction-Onion-Family-Growing-Shallots-ebook/dp/B0141GOXQA/ref=sr_1_5?ie=UTF8&qid=1440030038&sr=8-5&keywords=the+onion+family

Live Long and Prosper!

Author Bio

Dueep Jyot Singh is a Management and IT Professional who managed to gather Postgraduate qualifications in Management and English and Degrees in Science, French and Education while pursuing different enjoyable career options like being an hospital administrator, IT,SEO and HRD Database Manager/ trainer, movie , radio and TV scriptwriter, theatre artiste and public speaker, lecturer in French, Marketing and Advertising, ex-Editor of Hearts On Fire (now known as Solstice) Books Missouri USA, advice columnist and cartoonist, publisher and Aviation School trainer, ex-moderator on Medico.in, banker, student councilor ,travelogue writer ... among other things!

One fine morning, she decided that she had enough of killing herself by Degrees and went back to her first love -- writing. It's more enjoyable! She already has 48 published academic and 14 fiction- in- different- genre books under her belt.

When she is not designing websites or making Graphic design illustrations for clients , she is browsing through old bookshops hunting for treasures, of which she has an enviable collection – including R.L. Stevenson, O.Henry, Dornford Yates, Maurice Walsh, De Maupassant, Victor Hugo, Sapper, C.N. Williamson, "Bartimeus" and the crown of her collection- Dickens "The Old Curiosity Shop," and "Martin Chuzzlewit" and so on... Just call her "Renaissance Woman") - collecting herbal remedies, acting like Universal Helping Hand/Agony Aunt, or escaping to her dear mountains for a bit of exploring, collecting herbs and plants and trekking.

Check out some of the other JD-Biz Publishing books

Gardening Series on Amazon

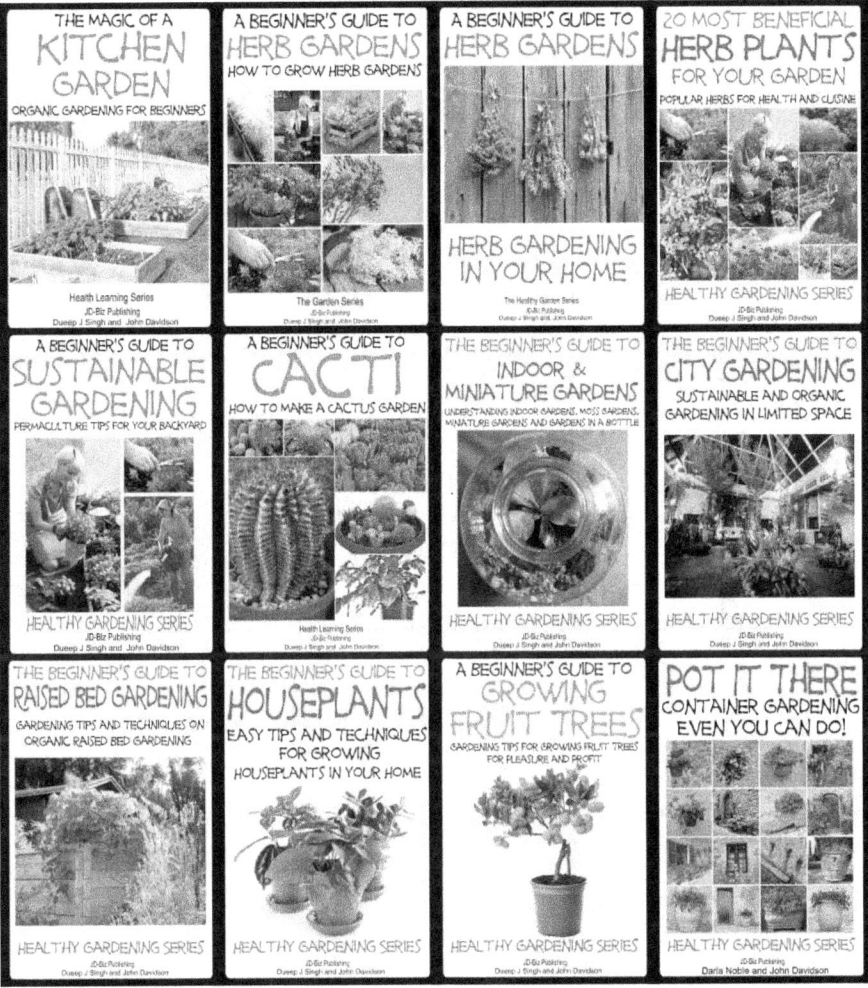

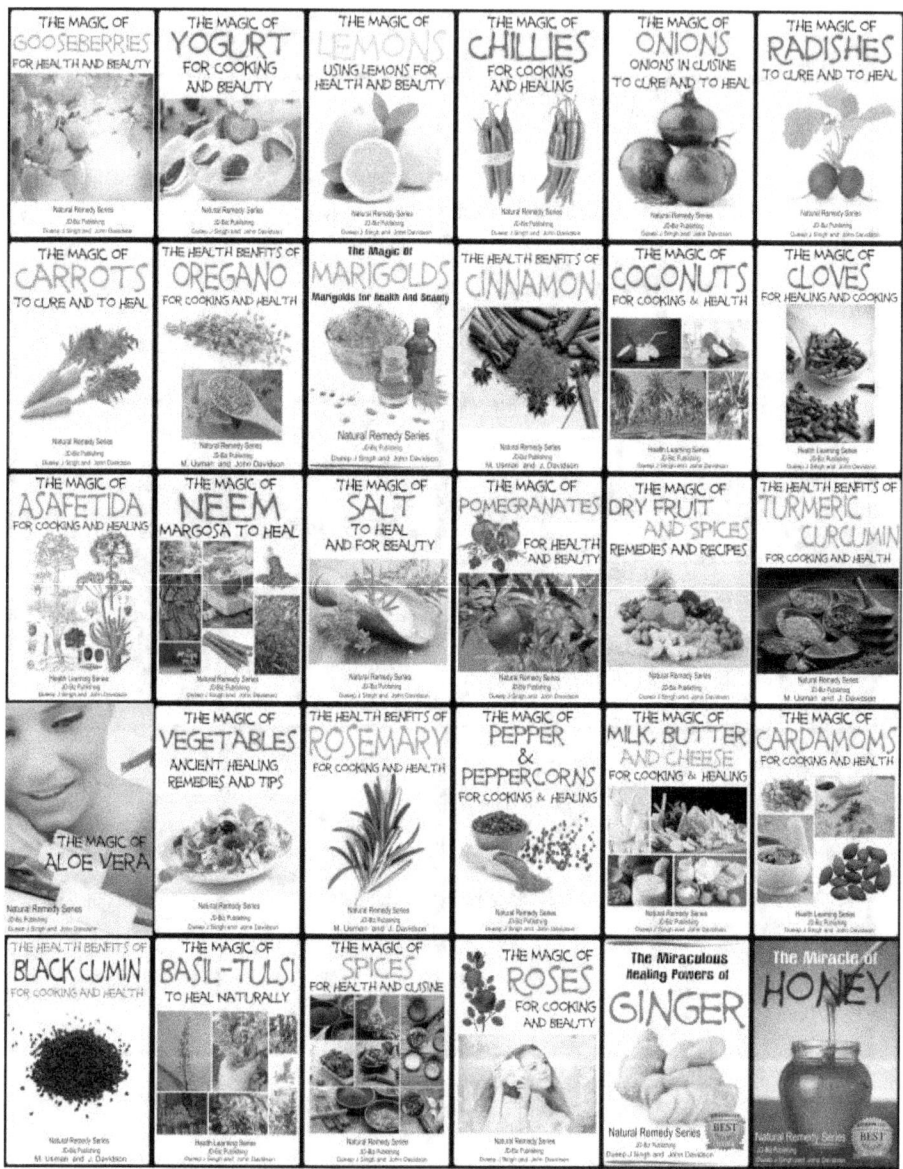

Country Life Books

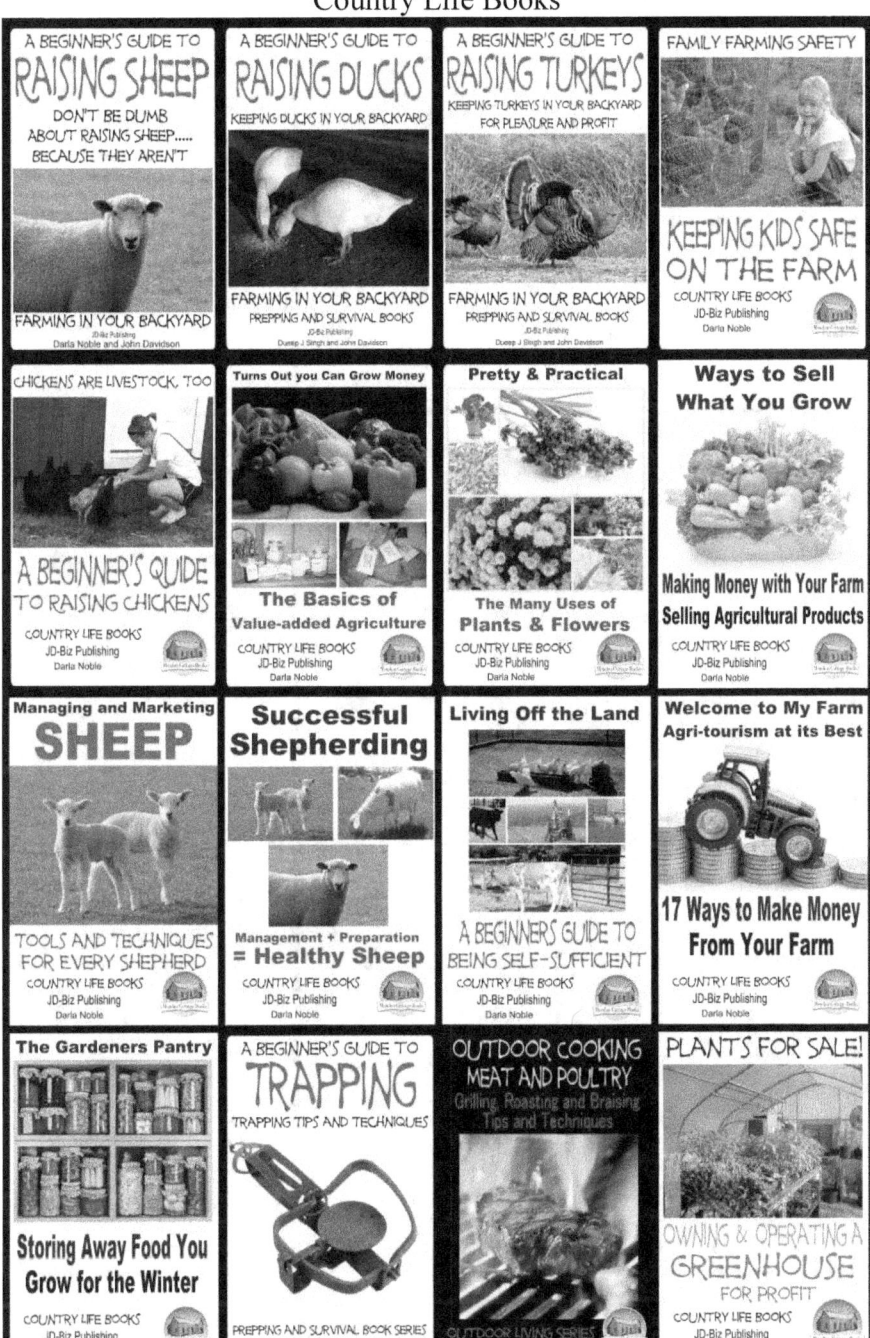

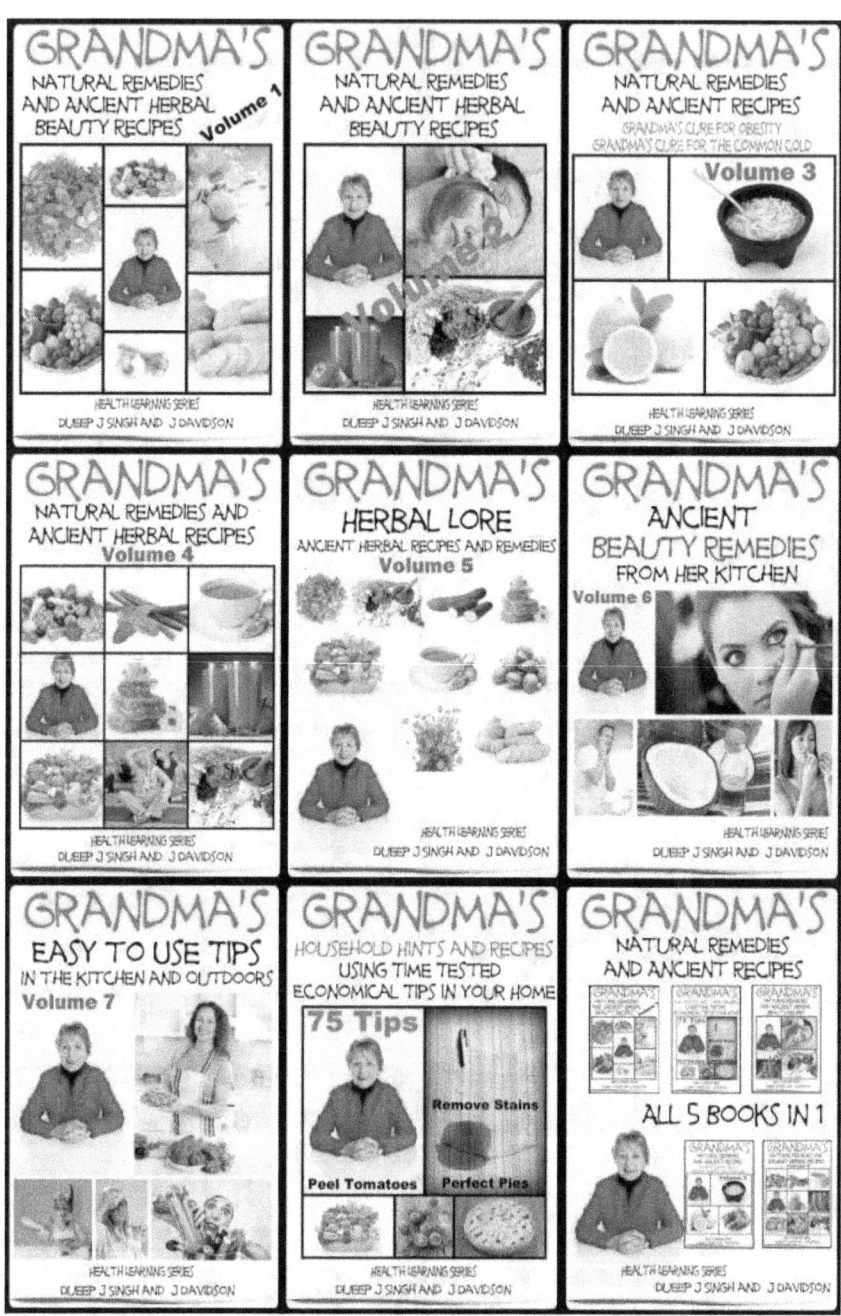

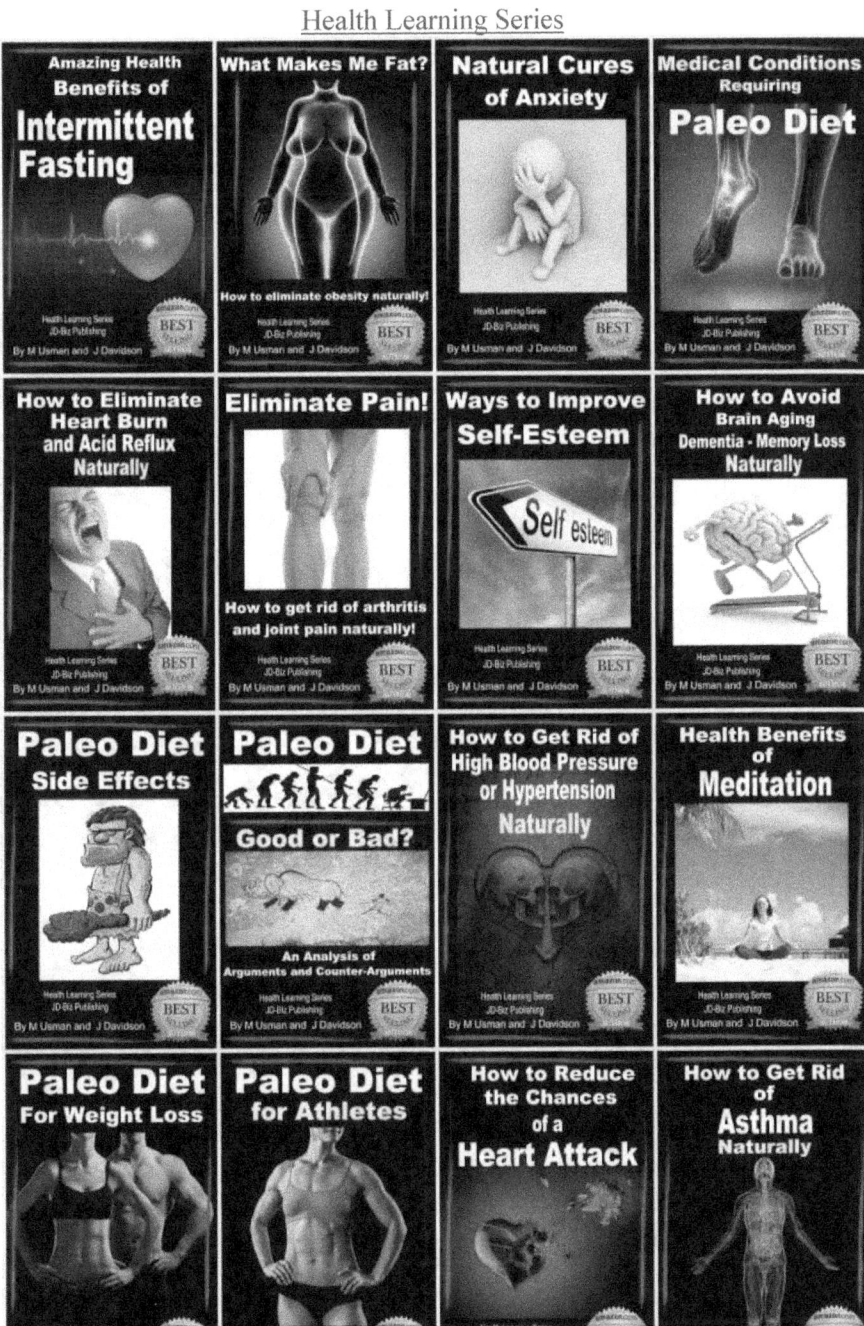

Amazing Animal Book Series

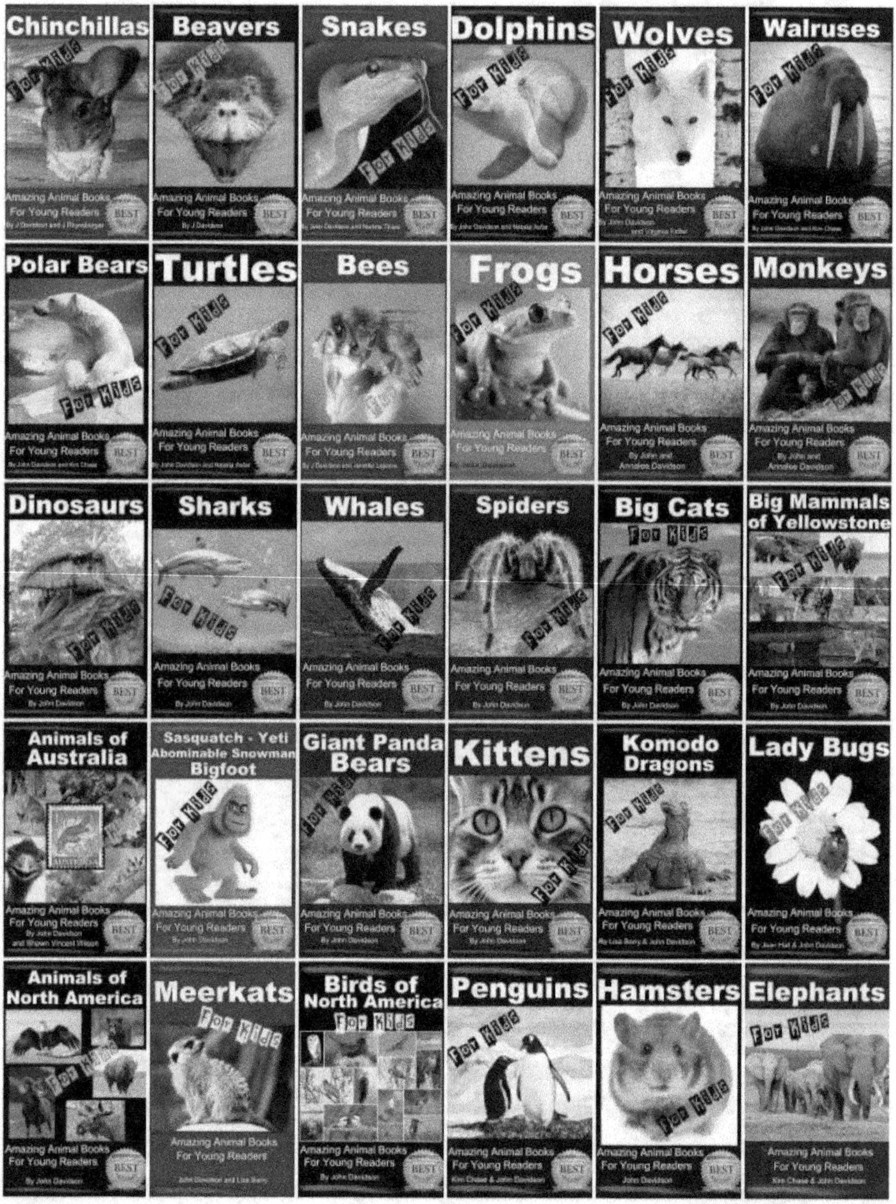

Learn To Draw Series

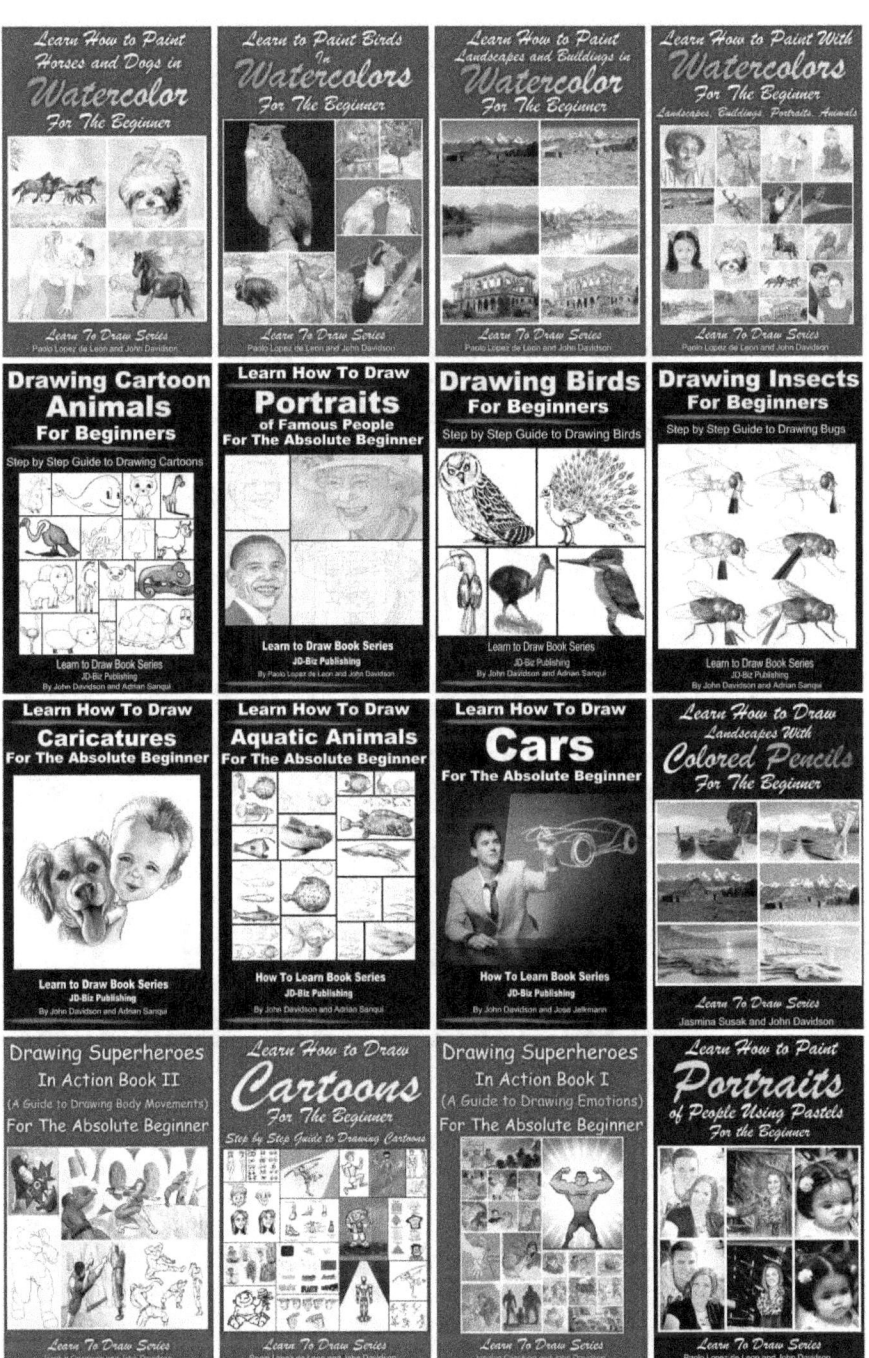

How to Build and Plan Books

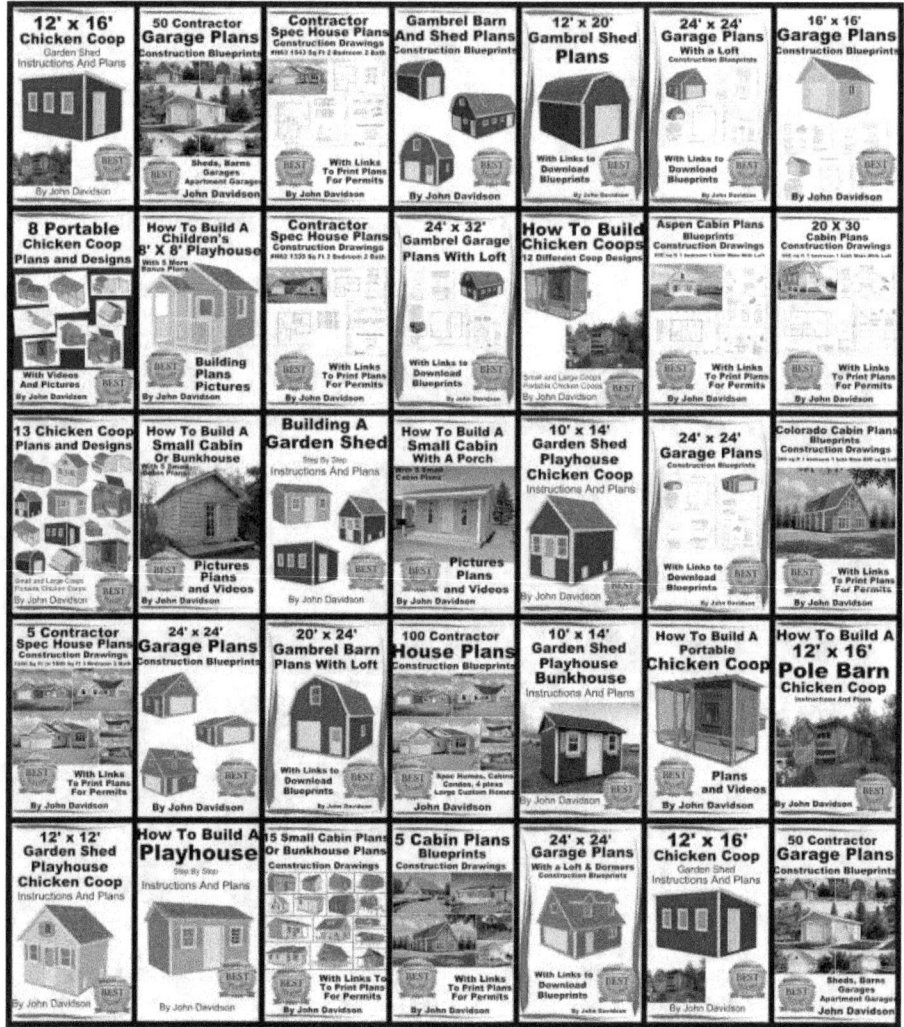

Entrepreneur Book Series

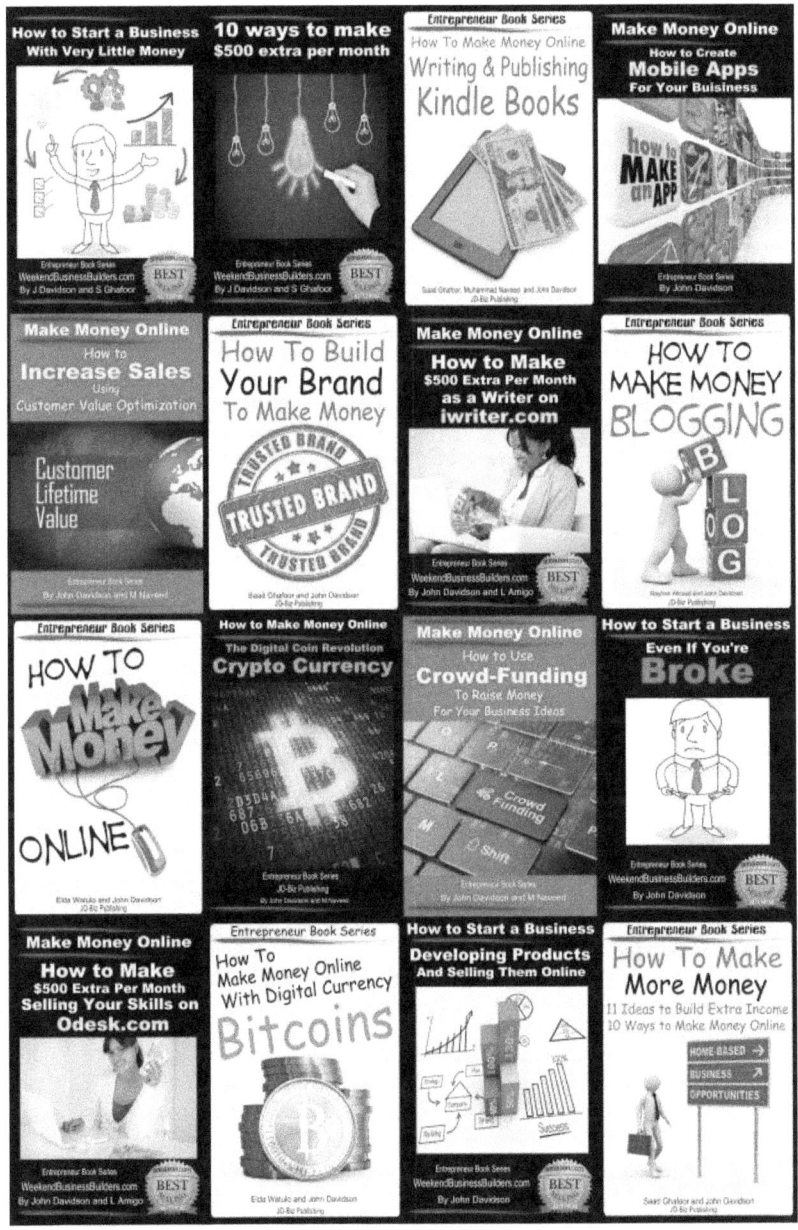

Our books are available at

1. Amazon.com

2. Barnes and Noble

3. Itunes

4. Kobo

5. Smashwords

6. Google Play Books

Publisher

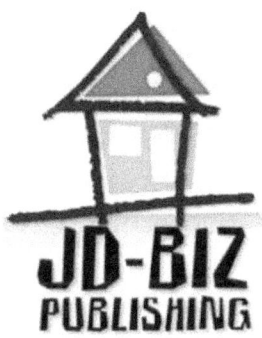

JD-Biz Corp

P O Box 374

Mendon, Utah 84325

http://www.jd-biz.com/

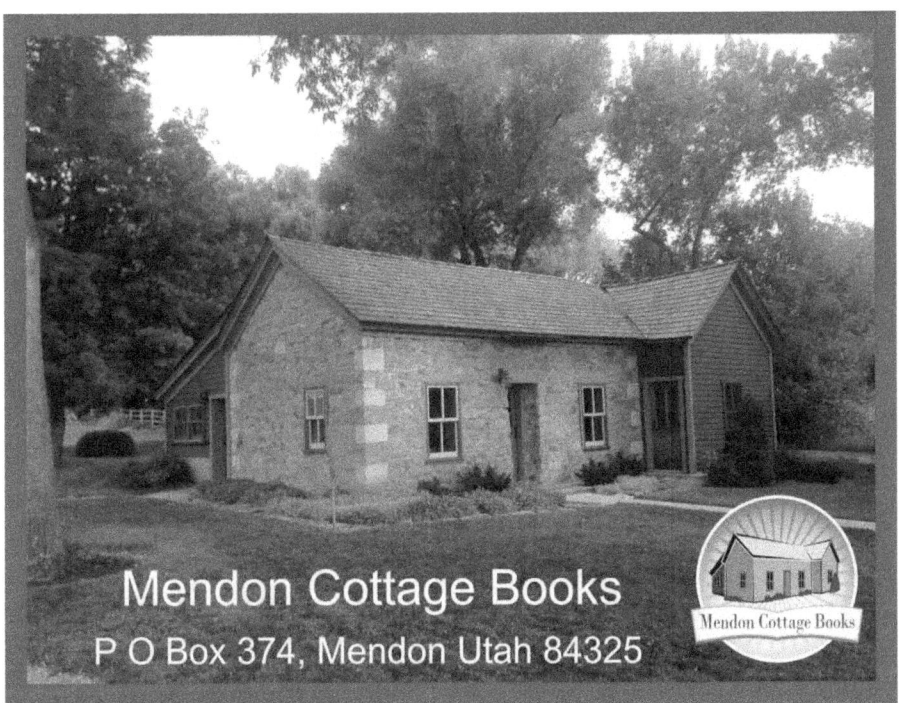

www.ingramcontent.com/pod-product-compliance
Lightning Source LLC
Chambersburg PA
CBHW070326290526
45791CB00003B/1272